What in the World are Prions?

Austin Mardon • Janvi Bedi • Ishpreet Chana • Rokya Harun
Jaime Johnson • Jess Jutras • Mehvish Masood • Ivan Quan •
Ivy Quan • Sapna Singh• Jessie Wang • Jonathan Wiebe

GM
PRESS

Typeset and cover design by Gillian Austin

ISBN: 978-1-77369-233-3

Golden Meteorite Press
#103, 11919 82 St NW
Edmonton, AB T5B 2W3
www.goldenmeteoritepress.com

GM
PRESS

"To scientific investigation that
creates new knowledge,
erases ignorance,
eradicates prejudice,
prevents disease,
alleviates suffering,
and enhances well-being"

—*Stanley B. Prusiner 2014*

Table of Contents

What in the World are Prions?

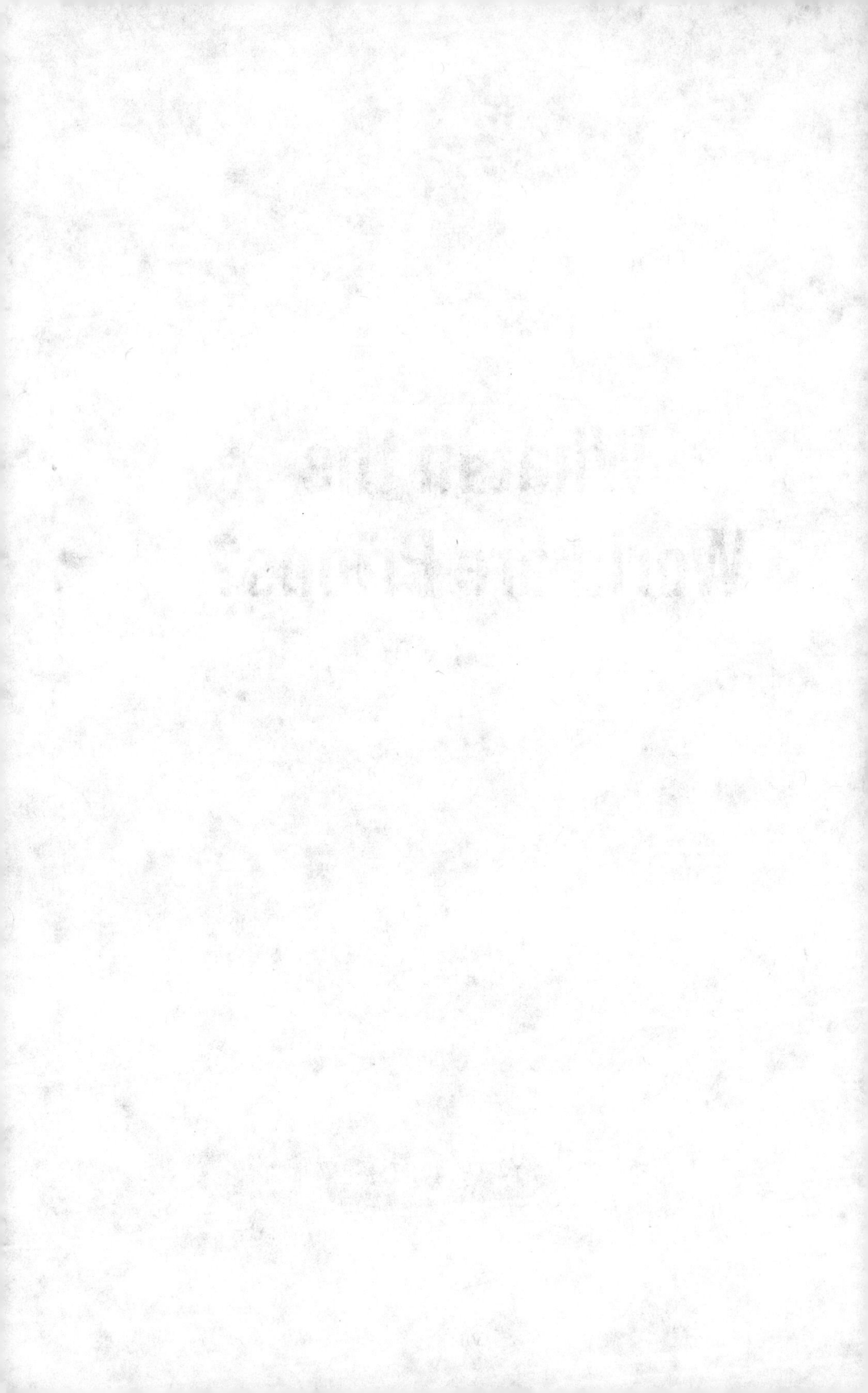

CHAPTER 1
Historical background of prions: a view from afar
JONATHAN WIEBE

One of the most unexpected and controversial findings in the field of medicine in the past 50 years were the identification of prions: misfolded proteins that act as pathogens, with the ability to bend and misshape other proteins to spread fatal diseases. The discovery of the prion in the 80s broke the rules of how diseases spread and replicated, flying in the face of the medical dogma of the time and taking years of experiments and studies before finally being accepted by the general scientific community (Zabel & Reid, 2015). Despite being a finding close to 40 years old at this point, much is still left to be understood about the prion, including how exactly it replicates and causes other proteins to fold, the origin of the deadly molecule itself, and - most pressingly - how to treat or cure any of the number of terminal diseases it causes in animals and humans.

The name 'prion' was coined by Dr. Stanley Prusiner, deriving from the words protein and infection, and is short for 'proteinaceous infectious particle.' Prions are best known as the believed cause of prion diseases, or Transmissible spongiform encephalopathies (TSEs), a group of fatal and often rapidly progressing neurodegenerative conditions affecting both humans and animals. Included in this group are diseases such as Scrapie in sheep, Chronic Wasting Disease (CWD) in deer, Bovine Spongiform Encephalopathy (BSE) or 'Mad Cow Disease' in bovine, and Creutzfeldt-Jakob Disease (CJD) in people (CDC, 2018). Though all known prion diseases are fatal, the protein that prions derive from - called cellular prion protein - are actually normally found in healthy bodies, primarily on cells in the central nervous system (Robertson, 2021). What sets this variant of cellular prion protein apart from its benign, everyday counterpart is its abnormal folded shape and its ability to induce this same abnormal folding in other proteins. The latter trait is also what makes prions stand out against other pathogens: rather than replicating inside the host through the use of nucleic acids like all other known infectious agents, the prion instead acts as a template and causes healthy proteins present in the host to bend and fold into the same abnormal form. As fascinating as this difference is, it is also this partially understood, but seemingly wholly unique mechanism of transmission that has contributed greatly to our long-time inability to adequately combat prions and prion diseases. In addition to the difficulties it causes for attempts at treatment today, this uniqueness is largely why it took so long for prions to be identified. Although we have only been directly studying and working against prions for the past 40 years, the history of prions and our exposure to their diseases extends centuries before they were ever named or even hypothesized.

The identification and description of proteins as distinct biological molecules was as early as the late 18th century by a French chemist named Antoine Fourcroy (Tanford & Reynolds, 2001). Although they were already known at this time to play an important role in cellular functions, proteins would not receive their name for another 50 years, when a Dutch chemist named Gerhardus Johannes Mulder characterized them and John Jakobs Berzelius suggested the name 'protein' in a correspondence with Mulder, after the word 'prota,' meaning 'of primary importance' in Greek (Tanford & Reynolds, 2001; Zabel & Reid, 2015). After this, it would still be yet another 40 years before Ferdinard Cohn classified bacteria and Robert Koch determined anthrax was caused by a bacterium (Zabel & Reid, 2015). Though it would still be nearly a century after this point before prions would first be proposed as the hypothetical infectious agent of Scrapie, and slightly longer still before prions were actually identified, by this point in time in the late 19th century humans had already been dealing with the first identified prion disease - Scrapie, found in sheep - for a century, and it would only be a few decades longer before we were introduced to the first known to affect humans.

Though Scrapie was first recorded at least as early as 1732, when observations of a disease causing Merino sheep to behave abnormally and excessively lick and scrape themselves raw against fences were made (Zabel & Reid, 2015), the exact origins and earliest cases of it are unknown. While it is entirely possible that scrapie has always affected sheep in small numbers, never quite managing to spread enough to get the attention of shepherds in times before the first written record of it, what is known with much greater certainty is that there was an increase in incidences of scrapie during the 18th and 19th centuries which coincided with the exportation of sheep from Spain (Duke University, n.d.......). At the time though, next to nothing was known about the strange disease affecting sheep, other than that it was known to be infectious within and amongst sheep, but humans could eat the infected sheep without any identifiable harm (Duke University, n.d.). As such, for the time being there was no need to look any further for a solution or a source - not that it was likely one could be found at the time since, as already mentioned, it would still be a century before proteins were identified, let alone named. Unfortunately, by the time the 19th and then early 20th century came and passed, the scientific community was not in much better of a position to treat or even identify the culprit behind scrapie, despite their advances in the understanding of how viruses and most other pathogens used information stored in their nucleic acid to replicate. The difference at this point though, nearly two centuries after the first recorded case of scrapie, was that people were about to have their first and, only a short while later, second run-ins with prion diseases that killed more than just sheep.

Due to the state of scientific understanding at the time, and the achievements regarding our understanding of viruses and how they replicate that would be made in the following few decades, the scientific community was in no position to identify the protein responsible for prion diseases. In fact, in 1920 when neurologists Hans Gerhard Creutzfeldt and Alfons Maria Jakob identified what would later be named CJD, scientists were at a loss (Zabel & Reid, 2015). With early theories that scrapie was caused by a 'slow virus' - a virus with a long incubation period before progressing or showing signs - it became increasingly unlikely that anyone would begin to look in the right direction for the cause of scrapie and CJD. Over the next 20 to 30 years scientists would make discovery after discovery about the nature of viruses and viral nucleic acids which, when combined with the slightly earlier theories about the origin of scrapie, directed the first theories of the cause of TSEs towards a 'slow virus.' By the time Sigurðsson (1954) too proposed that a slow virus was responsible for scrapie in sheep, scientists were no closer to the identification of the prion and the world was beginning to see the first few cases of the next prion disease to be found in humans: Kuru. In fact, by the time the first cases of Kuru were reported, it could be argued that scientists may have actually been further from identifying the cause of TSEs than before, due to a clue overlooked a decade earlier. In 1944 a veterinarian named W.S..... Gordon missed that, after using formalin to inactivate a virus in sheep tissue and using the newly treated tissue to vaccinate other sheep, these sheep became infected with scrapie that was unknowingly present in the treated tissue, killing the vaccinated sheep two years later and showing that methods that inactivate viruses had no effect on scrapie (Zabel & Reid, 2015).

With the identification of Kuru and the subsequent trip to Papua New Guinea in 1957 by American physician Carleton Gajdusek to investigate the strange disease (Duke University, n.d.), scientists were no closer to understanding any of the three prion diseases identified by this time. However, just two years after this trip collaborative efforts made by Gajdusek and other scientists revealed that Kuru, scrapie, and CJD were related, and in reality all different forms of the same neuropathy (Zabel & Reid, 2015). Unfortunately, neither these findings nor the recent experiments at the time exploring how scrapie was transmitted went much further for some time, as scientists then proposed that Kuru was caused by a slow virus, like how they thought scrapie and CJD were. Shortly after, scientists found what they thought was additional support for the slow virus theory of scrapie when a gene that seemed to control scrapie incubation periods in some mice was identified (Dickinson et al., 1968), and it seemed like progress towards the identification of the prion may be impeded again. Despite this outcome, the importance of the work done up to that point can't be understated, and while the first propositions of a protein pathogen were still roughly a decade off, progress had been made and the breakthrough stimulated further work on Kuru and the other prion diseases (Duke University, n.d.). In fact, in the years that followed the discovery of the relation between the prion diseases, and at that point two decades after Gordon missed that scrapie was not inactivated like other viruses would be, numerous scientists began to explore the stability of scrapie, and tried various experiments and a whole range of methods to inactivate scrapie (Zabel & Reid, 2015). In just a few years, it would be experiments like these that would lead a few scientists to develop theories which would contradict the biological dogma of the time itself.

As the experiments attempting to inactivate the scrapie agent continued and continued to fail, some scientists began to develop what were nearly heretical theories about the origin of the scrapie agent; what if instead of a slow virus, or a virus of any kind, as the cause of scrapie, the agent was instead of protein origin (Zabel & Reid, 2015)? One of the first major findings that led to this line of thinking was an experiment by Tikvah Alper and others (1967), where Alper, through her attempts to use ionizing radiation to inactivate the scrapie agent, discovered that high amounts of radiation failed to easily inactivate it, leading her to wonder if the scrapie agent replicated without the use of nucleic acid. Shortly after, others contributed further evidence to the idea that the scrapie agent was of protein origin through their experiments attempting to isolate the agent in tissue treated with formalin (Zabel & Reid, 2015). As important as these developments were, it was biophysicist John Griffith who first took it a step further, publishing

4

a paper speculating that the agent was protein in nature, and offering three hypothetical mechanisms of how a protein could be the cause of the diseases: the protein could be governed by a suppressed gene that is reactivated when the protein is introduced to the body, creating a process that resembles replication; the protein agent could be an abnormal form of a protein found regularly in the body, that then converts other proteins; or that the agent was an antibody that targeted itself, causing more of itself to be produced (Griffith, 1967) - with this last hypothesis being deemed least likely by Griffith at the time since no immune response was detected (Bolton, 2004). However, despite the work of others that followed Griffith's speculations, which continued to provide evidence suggesting the scrapie agent was of protein origin, the major turning point for prion research didn't come until nearly 20 years later when, in 1982, the prion would isolated and inactivated for the first time (Zabel & Reid, 2015).

In 1982, Stanley Prusiner pushed Griffith's work to a new level when Prusiner coined the term prion as a name for the hypothesized scrapie agent, and again later when he and others isolated and inactivated a prion (Zabel & Reid, 2015). Although Griffith's second hypothesis - that the prion is an abnormal form of a cellular protein - has formed the basis for prion theory for several decades now, when the prion was first identified it was Griffith's first hypothesis - that the prion production was controlled by a normally dormant gene - that gained favor by many scientists. This was largely due to the fact that, when first discovered, it did not seem that prions were present in healthy individuals, only infected ones. However, when it was discovered that prions existed in healthy individuals in a different and harmless form, Griffith's second hypothesis was adopted (Bolton, 2004). Despite these findings, it still took quite some time before the general scientific community accepted the prion, or 'protein only,' hypothesis (Zabel & Reid, 2015). But the evidence kept mounting, and in the years that followed Prusiner's isolation of the prion scientists continued to perform experiments and broaden our understanding of the prion, and of how a protein could function as a pathogen, to the point where few now would deny that normal cellular prion protein can be misfolded into the pathological form, causing prion diseases. Over the ensuing years though, one particularly interesting source of support for the prion hypothesis was yeast of all things (Zabel & Reid, 2015). Through his work with yeast, Reed Wickner, M.D. (1994) discovered two altered forms of proteins in yeast, which he determined to be analogous to prions, and proposed that the production of these two prions was essentially the yeast's last ditch attempt to survive off of poor nitrogen sources. Although likely not a place scientists expected to find supporting evidence for the prion hypothesis, Wickner's work provided much needed corroboration of prions as a biological paradigm and, further still, presented an easy way to rapidly generate prions for study, ultimately accelerating their study and greatly informing the research into those prions found in people and animals (Zabel & Reid, 2015).

As great and, in the case of the last example, surprising as much of the research following Prusiner's isolation and inactivation of the prion was, the years shortly following the work of Prusiner and others unfortunately brought more than just progress. Although no great works or discoveries were made that led people away from progressing prion research in the years that followed - as we have seen happen at a few different times in the long and winding history of the prion - the world was unfortunately introduced to yet another new prion disease: Bovine Spongiform Encephalopathy (BSE), better known as Mad Cow Disease. As early as in 1986, Mad Cow Disease, as BSE had begun to be called by that point, had become a significant health concern (Duke University, n.d.). It was determined that the disease was being spread through the cattle by their feed, which contained brain tissue from other prion infected herd members, leading to restrictions being placed on the content of feed. However, only a decade after the initial Mad Cow Disease outbreak, a failure to properly uphold regulations and follow precautions in British slaughterhouses led to cases of a variant of CJD which affected a much younger population.

Upon further investigation by later studies, it was suspected that this variant of CJD came from an Antelope imported to a British safari park from South America in the 70s; from there, it is believed that eventually the infected antelope was ground into cattle feed, spreading these new prions to the cows, and from them to us (Duke University, n.d.). This laxness ultimately led to a 10 year ban by the European Union on the import of British beef, and, more significantly, the introduction of variant CJD (vCJD) into humans (Duke University, n.d.). Thankfully, though the variant disease killed 165 people in Britain and caused a great deal of fear amongst the public, the rates of infection for the disease were not as high as it was first thought they would be (Duke University, n.d.). This, it turned out, was due to the fact that in order for vCJD to spread in a person, that individual needed to have a particular pre-existing mutation in the gene for cellular prion protein - a mutation only 40% of the population has (Brown et al., 2001). Nevertheless, the introduction of vCJD led to the British Government killing herds of cattle that had the greatest risk of getting Mad Cow Disease in an attempt to prevent further spread (Duke University, n.d.). Unfortunately, for the most part the damage was done, as Mad Cow Disease began appearing in herds around the globe, beginning with herds in France in 2000, then herds in the remaining countries from the EU shortly after, and then, before long, herds in Canada and the United States (Duke University, n.d.).

For the most part, this brings us up to date on the broader history of the prion. Though it took some time to identify the prion, and longer still to accumulate enough evidence to sway the broader scientific community, the prion hypothesis is now widely accepted as the explanation for what causes TSEs and how they spread. The things that make the prion so unique as a pathogen are also largely what made identifying them such a long and arduous process in the first place - as well as what makes dealing with them and the diseases they cause so difficult to this day. Now, though prions and their nearly 300 year history have been condensed and introduced here, there is much left to be discussed and learned about the prion. Scientists haven't stopped researching and pushing the bounds of what we know about prions, and advancements have been made since the spread of Mad Cow Disease and the introduction of vCJD in the late 20th/early 21st centuries - for all we know, progress towards a breakthrough could be being made at this very moment as this is being read. Though there is still much left to be learned about the prion, there is even more left unsaid - a wrong hopefully made right over the course of the remaining chapters. Throughout the rest of this book, a variety of areas related to the prion will be explored in greater depth than can be achieved in this chapter alone. From glimpses into what we know about the structure and function of the prion, to explorations of where the research is headed and what we are still trying to figure out, the remainder of this book aims to provide comprehensive summaries of numerous topics surrounding the prion - beginning in the next chapter with a look at the person who found and named the prion.

8

CHAPTER 2
Stanley B. Prusiner

JESS JUTRAS

Stanley B. Prusiner is a distinguished neurologist and biochemist. His long-term research in neurodegenerative diseases has advanced scientific knowledge of diseases like Creutzfeldt-Jakob Disease (CJD), Alzheimer's disease, and Parkinson's disease. Prusiner and colleagues have studied and are currently studying causes, biologies of, and treatments for fatal neurodegenerative diseases. Prior to studying neurology and infectious diseases, Prusiner studied Latin, philosophy, history of architecture, economics, and Russian history (1997). His familial background likely inspired these subjects. His paternal grandfather immigrated to Sioux City, Iowa, United States, from Russia as a young child. His father and grandfather resided there, among a tight-knit community of Russian Jewish immigrants (1997). After a career with the US Naval, his father moved Prusiner and his mother from Des Moines, Iowa to Cincinnati, Ohio, where he worked as an architect (1997, 2017).

Prusiner completed a BA in Chemistry and an MD from the University of Pennsylvania (2017), where he also researched hypothermia with Sidney Wolfson in the Department of Surgery (1997). Additionally, Prusiner worked with Britton Chance, a pioneer in biomedical optics research and a pronounced member of the scientific community (UPenn, n.d.), and Olov Lindberg of the Wenner-Gren Institute in Stockholm (1997), with adipocytes or adipose tissue, a lipid (aka fat). Soon after, he worked for the National Institute of Health (NIH) under Earl Stadtman, studying glutaminase in *E. coli* (1997). Prusiner's three years as a lieutenant commander in the US Public Health Service at the NIH developed his research skills and set him on the path of a neurology residency (1997, 2017).

In 1972, Prusiner was a neurology resident at the University of California, San Francisco. Here, he encountered a patient dying after two months of becoming ill of CJD. Her brain degenerated rapidly while her body stayed intact, unaffected by the disease. Prusiner (1998) reported that the patient experienced no fever response, no increase in white blood cells (WBCs) or cell count, and no antibody protection or humoral immune response (pp. 13363). The results of Prusiner's patient discourse sparked his interest in neurodegenerative diseases and led to his discovery of Prions, proteinaceous infectious particles or proteins with no nucleic acid (13363, 13365).

Prions are infectious pathogens that cause fatal neurodegenerative diseases, which can present as genetic, infectious, or sporadic disorders. All mammals have protein cells; prion diseases modify the prion protein (PrP). Prusiner's concept of the prion can explain how heritable diseases can also be infectious and defines how the PrP modifies.

However, Prusiner did not discover prions without barriers. He studied neuro-degenerative diseases, or "slow virus" diseases (a name Prusiner considered "misleading" (pp. 86)), assays in mice and hamsters, and scrapie agents for many years -- the incubation periods for these diseases are two years or longer (2014) -- with the assistance of multiple funding programs including the NIH. The more he studied scrapie anticipating a virus, the more he discovered that the protein was devoid of nucleic acids, a key component in viruses. As the data accumulated, Prusiner (1997) became increasingly confident that he had discovered something unique about neurodegenerative diseases.

After publishing his first article introducing his hypothesis naming prions, a windstorm of backlash came at him. Claiming that prions can spread infection without deoxyribonucleic acid (DNA) or ribonucleic acid (RNA) went against a "central dogma of biology" (pp. 85) that DNA was "essential for *all* reproduction" (2007, italics added); his definition and theory were scientific heresy in the community (pp. 133). Although skeptics not only tried to disprove his theories using scientific methods but also attempted to viciously attack Prusiner personally (1997), he continued researching prions and their modifications. With the support of his family and the help of a team of colleagues, he overcame the controversy and continued crucial scientific work that had not been done before.

By the early 1990s, Prusiner, Leroy Hood, Charles Weissmann, George Carlson, David Kingsbury, Stephen DeArmond, Ruth Gabizon, Karen Hsiao, Michael

Scott, and Fred Cohen had all contributed to the acceptance of the prion theories. Although there were still grey areas, for instance, what specifically caused normal PrP to convert into its "disease-causing form" (1997), Prusiner had advanced the scientific knowledge of this malicious pathogen tenfold. For his many years of effort, prions became more widely accepted among scientists, and he won many scientific awards, including the Nobel Prize in Physiology or Medicine (1997). No one could describe Prusiner's (2014) arduous journey as well as he has in his own book, Madness and Memory: The Discovery of Prions--a New Biological *Principle of Disease*, a "first-person account of the thinking, the experiments, and the surrounding events that led to the identification" of prions (x).

Since discovering the intricacies of prions and their ability to misfold healthy proteins into diseased cells, Prusiner (2014) and colleagues have discovered that prions not only affect CJD, kuru, and scrapie agents but also play an essential role in other neurodegenerative diseases such as Parkinson's disease and Alzheimer's disease. Prusiner's concepts and research have been at the forefront of health discussions (2014), including the long-running international health issue of "mad cow disease" from 1986 to 2012 (n.d.). He is still at the head of health discussions; especially recently (2017), while researching treatment for other degenerative nervous-system diseases (2014) in partnership with Alzheon, Inc. Alzheon is a bio-pharmaceutical company "focused on developing new medicines for patients suffering from Alzheimer's disease and other neurological and psychiatric disorders" (2017). As Guy McKhann observes in his review of Prusiner's book, Prusiner has again steered research and opinion to an undiscovered realm of neurodegenerative diseases despite battling consistent skepticism and criticism (2014). The BrightFocus Foundation, a prominent research funding non-profit organization, says, "Dr. Prusiner's research may one day lead to a treatment and cure for Alzheimer's," and possibly even more fatal neurodegenerative diseases (n.d.). Prusiner has voiced many thanks to BrightFocus and all other funding programs for presenting the opportunities he needed to propel science forward (2016).

The backlash against Prusiner's Prion definition and findings

After submitting his landmark article to Science (and before it was published), Prusiner presented his findings briefly at the Fifth International Congress of Virology in Strasbourg, France (2014). Although he did not dare name prions (he would wait until his article was published), he broke the news of his "infectious proteinaceous particle" (2014) and was met with disbelief and hostility (pp. 88).

11

Questions arose ranging from predictable: "How can a virus be only protein?" "How can it be devoid of nucleic acid?" to deeming Prusiner inept: "How can anyone who calls himself a scientist not find a nucleic acid core?" "Finding evidence for a nucleic acid is easy. You must have done something wrong!" (pp. 88). Despite his many years of devout research, his team of highly esteemed experts, and his conclusive evidence, scientific critics and common-folk skeptics alike refused to acknowledge the brilliance of Prusiner's findings.

Prusiner battled a long wait and editor tirades before *Science* published the article as had been promised. The push came when Frank Sooy asked for David Perlman, a reporter for the *San Francisco Chronicle*, to be allowed early access to Prusiner's article. Perlman published his story (2014), talking about a "Weird new form of life" that Prusiner discovered while giving few details (pp. 91-2). The pressure was put on Science to finally publish Prusiner's article, despite their fear of causing commotion and disruption (which, as aforementioned, is what happened). Despite Prusiner (2014) providing the previous academic work that had been done on diseases like CJD and kuru by scientists Bill Hadlow, C. Joseph Gibbs and D. Carleton Gajdusek, Raymond Latarjet and Tikvah Alper, that assisted Prusiner in developing his theories, critics refused to believe that there were no nucleic acids present (pp. 93). Despite having presented years of research and findings that separated viruses from scrapie agents and breaking ground in neurodegenerative disease knowledge, Prusiner was described as "impulsive, presumptuous, reckless, ambitious, aggressive, callous, manipulative, and egotistical" (pp. 93). In reality, he was a determined scientist and investigator who had taken an interest in truly helping treat and cure fast working and fatal diseases of the brain.

The scientific community had the right to be skeptical of such a bold claim; they do not experience breakthroughs and "big new ideas" often (pp. 94). However, no matter where Prusiner went, whether it to a lecture, press conference, or interview, he faced considerable push-back against his evidence and claims (pp. 94). Each conversation tended to repeat arguments he had already made and continued down an unproductive path. Despite him and his family (especially his wife) becoming increasingly stressed with the negative media coverage, Prusiner remained objective and resolute. He and the colleagues who supported his efforts continued to produce vital research and evidence that a virus was not the cause of scrapie and CJD (pp. 94).

Even after working closely with Ted Diener (2014), who discovered viroids (small, highly infectious RNAs), using the viroids as a control, and concluding that prions were not viruses nor viroids, the debate rampaged on (pp. 95). Their published work in *Proceedings of the National Academy of Sciences*, "Viroids and Prions," did not allay critics' suspicions that scrapie was caused by a virus with a small nucleic acid (pp. 95). Prusiner and his research team spent years thereafter continuing to search for the "mythical nucleic acid of the prion," occasionally finding some evidence for it and subsequently debunking the finding with further examinations and tests (pp. 95-6). If there were nucleic acids to be found, Prusiner would be the one to find it and continue from there. However, none were found, and he has been able to continue his prion research to date.

While asking himself why there was such resistance to his concepts (2014), Prusiner thought back to 1944 when Oswald Avery, Colin MacLeod, and Maclyn McCarty discovered evidence that DNA composed a "transforming principle" (pp. 96). It had taken 75 years from Friedrich Miescher's isolation of DNA for those three distinguished investigators to confirm their findings. It then took over a decade for nucleic acid to be accepted as genetic material (pp. 96). Relating the controversy and slow acceptance of DNA to his own concepts of prions, Prusiner quotes Belgian playwright Maurice Maeterlinck: "At every crossway on the road that leads to the future, tradition has placed, against each of us, ten thousand men to guard the past" (pp. 96).

During his long-term "joust" with the press, Prusiner experienced a problem that exists with all media coverage, especially in scientific and academic communities (pp. 143-152). The more he talked to them, the less likely it was that the *truth* would spread about his hard work and incredible findings. His intention to inform the general public of new research discoveries in his field by speaking to interested reporters (pp. 142-3) morphed into him feeling betrayed and hopeless (pp. 147, 149). Thankfully, the derogative attacks on Prusiner's character and research ironically belied the support he gained from scientists in and out of the scrapie field. Prusiner decided not to discuss his science with the press any longer so as not to cause "conjecture and speculation" that were of no value to the real progress he was making in his field and instead continued to "produce data and let the published record in refereed scientific journals speak for itself" (pp.149). So, he let the critics stay "stuck in one little framework," as Douglas J. Lanska (2018) put it in his interview with Prusiner, while Prusiner continued to work toward bigger and better ideas.

Supporters and acceptance of Prusiner's Prion concepts

Prusiner was not solely contested. He encountered many strong scientists, researchers, and academics that supported and continue to support his work. Lanska is one of these people. Lanska's and Lauren E. Klaffke's private and public interview with Prusiner in Boston for the American Academy of Neurology Oral History Project encapsulates the support he had (2017). These three had genuine chemistry that portrayed the truths behind Prusiner's background, research, and the battle he has fought to be recognized as having an earnest and profound scientific discovery. Apart from his struggles, they discussed a wide range of topics, including a friendly mention of Prusiner's trip to the South Sandwich Islands where he visited Prion Island -- the home of the prion (pronounced PRY-on) bird, the main competitor of Prusiner's name choice for prions (pp. 7-9). They discussed the aforementioned opportunities Wolfson, Chance, and others granted Prusiner -- opportunities that changed Prusiner's life from one with no real direction or desire to one packed full of ambition to solve problems and help people along the way (pp. 14-8). Prusiner was never interested in "becoming a billionaire" or acquiring fame; he was only interested in doing research and living a healthy life spending his time attempting to allow others the chance to live healthy lives (pp. 19-20).

As Lanska observed, since discovering what he wanted to accomplish, Prusiner focused on and refused to stray from his concepts. He "pulled colleagues in ... built collaborations," solved problems like nobody's business, and succeeded in "accomplish[ing] something that seemed impossible to accomplish" (pp. 22). Prusiner dedicates his successful career (to his plentiful opportunities and) to "wonderful luck" (pp. 26). Prusiner is a man full of gratitude and appreciation for a life well-led. He has put his skills and knowledge to the forefront of neuro-degenerative brain disease cures and treatments and will continue his ground-breaking research until he can no longer. As the scientific community has come slowly around to (for the most part) accepting Prusiner's evidenced concept of prions, so has the general public. The world is a better place because of Stanley B. Prusiner's revolutionary ideas.

CHAPTER 3
Importance of Prions

ROKYA HARUN

Prions are infectious pathogens composed of misfolded proteins found in human and animal brains and other tissues (Telling, 2013). The discovery of prions has been significant because they challenge the idea of the Central Dogma principle in molecular biology due to the fact that prions do not contain any genetic material (RNA or DNA), and yet are still capable of self-replicating (Bruner, 2020). The Central Dogma states that nucleic acids, used to form RNA and DNA molecules, should only have the ability to self-replicate (Bruner 2020). Despite not having nucleic acids, prions can still be transmitted like infectious organisms, such as viruses and bacteria (Colorado State University, n.d.). Prions acquire the ability to transmit when an infectious prion acts as a template to change the normal conformation of the host encoded prion protein into its infectious form (Telling, 2013). This type of conformational templating explains the general mechanism of information transfer via proteins and prion diseases (Telling, 2013). The pathogenic prion protein (PrP^{Sc}) is a distorted version of the host encoded normal prion protein (PrP^{c}) (Teller, 2013). Although, according to the Alberta Prion Research Institute (n.d.), the precise function of the normal host encoded prion proteins is unknown, they have been found to partake in immune responses, cell to cell communications, copper transportation and the protection of cells from electro-chemical stress. It is important to research prions to determine their contributions to the current understanding of neurodegenerative disorders, identify their high resolution structures and related functions, detail their means of transmission between and across species, and learn about their role in the inheritance of phenotypic traits.

Prion Diseases and Transmission Barriers

Prion diseases must be studied to aid in the development of treatments for protein misfolding neurodegenerative diseases. Prion diseases are fatal neurodegenerative diseases that affect the health of animals and humans and are known as transmissible spongiform encephalopathies (TSEs) (Tittelmeier, J et al., 2020). Pathogenic prions can cause mad cow disease in cattle, chronic wasting disease (CWD) in deer and elk, scrapie in sheep and goats, and Creutzfeldt-Jakob disease (CJD) in humans (Tittelmeier, J et al., 2020). Prion diseases can arise spontaneously without any known cause, be acquired by infection or through inheritance (Collinge & Clarke, 2007). For example, according to Belay & Schonberger (2005), about 10%–15% of CJD cases occur as an autosomal dominant inherited disease caused by a pathogenic mutation of the PrP (prion) encoding gene. On the other hand, they reveal that about 85% of CJD cases occur spontaneously with no characteristic pattern of transmission. Belay & Schonberger (2005) explained that random mutations in somatic cells could facilitate the spontaneous generation of the self-replicating prions resulting in the sporadic etiology of CDC. Although prion diseases are rarely transmitted between individuals for humans, according to Belay & Schonberger (2005), three main external sources of infection pose a risk to human health. These include the iatrogenic transmission of CJD, the threat of exposure to BSE-contaminated cattle products leading to the occurrence of a variant Creutzfeldt-Jakob disease (vCJD) form, and the possible zoonotic transmission of CWD from elk and deer to humans (Belay & Schonberger, 2005). Despite the fact that human to human transmission of prion diseases is uncommon, they most likely form of this method of transmission is through iatrogenic or medical means involving the transfer of tissues from a human with an undiagnosed prion disease, such as those evident in donors of growth hormone therapy and tissue grafts from the brain to recipients (Colorado State University, n.d.). Prion diseases have also shown to transmit across species, such as the transfer of BSE from cattle to humans resulting in a newly formed human disease known as Variant Creutzfeldt-Jakob disease (vCJD) caused by human exposure to BSE-contaminated cattle products (Belay & Schonberger, 2005). In mammals, a wide range of misfolded 3D shapes or conformations are possible for prions, but only a subset of these conformations are compatible with each individual species' host encoded primary amino acid structure (Collinge & Clarke, 2007). The 3D conformation of the prion proteins is said to determine the stain's biological characteristics (Collinge & Clarke, 2007). How easily prions are transmitted between species is associated with the overlap of stable or allowed misfolded prion conformations from the different host encoded primary structures from the two species (Collinge & Clarke, 2007). For example, BSE can transmit efficiently across a range of intermediate species exhibiting distinct prion primary structures, all the while maintaining its biological characteristics, despite strain mutation, because the conformation of the BSE strain may be thermodynamically favored for a range of different species (Collinge & Clarke, 2007). This accounts for the cross-species pathogenicity of BSE. Taking into account differences in strains, the distinguished strain seen in CJD and vCJW are due to differences in prion conformation, resulting in disease-phenotype variability where varying disease characteristics may arise (Belay & Schonberger, 2005). For example, the variant of the Creutzfeldt-Jakob disease is distinguished from CJD by the younger median age of affected patients, its clinical and neuro-pathologic features, and the biochemical properties (Belay & Schonberger, 2005). As a result, the mechanism of prion propagation, determined by the prion strain and the host-tissue environment can help to explain prion disease pathogenesis (Collinge & Clarke, 2007). Although the transmission of prion diseases across species seems to be limited by an apparent "species barrier", since the propaga-tion of such prions requires overlap of prion conformations between species, the occurrence of BSE and its transmission to humans indicate that animal prion diseases can pose a significant public health risk (Belay & Schonberger, 2005). That is why the cross species transmission of CWD from deer and elk to humans is a potential concern. The transmission methods of prion diseases need to be expanded on to minimize the public health impact on humans, while finding ways to economically dispose of specified risk materials that have the ability to transmit prion diseases (Alberta Research Institute, n.d.).The Alberta Prion Research Institute (n.d.) explains that misfolded prions are unique in the way that they are able to transfer certain diseases within and between species by acting as an infectious agent, unlike any other misfolded proteins. Normally, the body can get rid of misfolded proteins; however, misfolded prions start to aggregate since they have the ability to convert normal neighbouring prions into misfolded prions also (Alberta Prion Research Institute, n.d.). The aggregation of these prions form large clusters known as fibrils, which then accumulate into plaques (Alberta Prion Research Institute, n.d.). A study by Acevedo-Morantes and Willie (2014) assessed the structural models of prions. They detailed that the structures of prions themselves are important in understanding prion diseases. They reviewed the various discovered prion related gene mutations, stating that certain mutations could directly affect prion structures and could explain the mechanism of prion conversion and replication into its pathogenic form. The structural changes that occur when the prions transform into their pathogenic form can alter their function and could be used to explain their toxicity and can, ultimately, be studied to understand prion diseases (Acevedo-Morantes & Willie, 2014).

Neurodegenerative Disorders and Molecular Chaperones

All prion diseases exhibit an accumulation of infectious prions (PrP^{Sc}) within the central nervous system of an animal (Tittelmeier et al., 2020). Normal host encoded prions (PrP^{C}) are cell membrane proteins that have the highest amount of expression within neurons of the brain and the spinal cord since these prions are thought to be involved in maintaining synapses and neuroprotective signaling (Tittelmeier et al., 2020). However, little is understood about how prion neurodegeneration causes cell death as they do not elicit an immune response in the host (Belay & Schonberger, 2005). Belay and Schonberger (2005) go onto to explain that although the mechanism of brain damage due to pathogenic prions is not greatly understood, the progression in neural accumulation of disease-associated prions may damage neurons directly while the reduced titre of normal prion proteins may interfere with their presumed function of neuroprotection from electrochemical stresses, thus contributing to further neurodegeneration. The structure of the misfolded PrP^{Sc} gives insight into the pathogenic mechanisms of prions. For instance, the "protein only hypothesis" states that the abnormal isoform (PrP^{Sc}) of the host-encoded cellular prion protein (PrP^{C}) is the main and possibly the only component of the transmissible agent or prion (Collinge & Clarke, 2007). However, the mechanism of this conformational transformation from PrP^{c} into PrP^{Sc} remains unclear and requires further research to uncover the high resolution structures of the prion isoforms (Teller, 2013). A journal article by Teller (2013) explained that PrP^{c} are predominantly α-helical, monomeric, protease-sensitive, and detergent-soluble. On the other hand, the disease-causing PrP^{Sc} are rich in beta-sheets, aggregation-prone, protease-resistant, and detergent-insoluble. Teller (2013) emphasized that the fundamental event resulting in the propagation of these prions was the physiochemical conversion of the PrP^{c} into PrP^{Sc}, where they differ in their monomer conformation and their ability to aggregate. The infectious prion proteins display an increase in beta sheets in their conformation, which lends them to form highly ordered amyloid fibrils or clusters (Tittelmeier et al., 2020). Collinge & Clarke (2007) explain that prions are presumed to be self-propagating amyloid forms of PrP^{c} in which the ends of the propagating clusters form the infectious entity, where fragmentation of the prions results in the exponential rise in prion concentration (Tittelmeier et al., 2020). This happens as the amyloid fibrils act as a template to misfold the normal protein monomer into the amyloid conformation and add onto the amyloid clusters. Tittelmeier et al. (2020) explains that these growing clusters of fibrils can accumulate and be deposited within and outside of cells, where the deposition patterns may be characteristic of their respective neurodegenerative disease. Although it has been established that the misfolding of prion proteins can cause prion diseases, it is also true that the accumulation of misfolded proteins (not prions) into amyloid deposits is characteristic of many age-related neurodegenerative diseases, including Alzheimer's disease (AD), Parkinson's disease (PD), Huntington's Disease (HD), and Amyotrophic Lateral Sclerosis (ALS) (Tittelmeier et al., 2020). For example, Alzheimer's disease, which is not a type of prion disease, is characterized by the misfolding of amyloid-β (Aβ) and Tau (MAPT) proteins (Tittelmeier et al., 2020). However, the similar characteristic of the presence of misfolded protein between diseases, such as Alzheimer's disease and prion diseases, show that it is important to research prions to develop a better understanding on the etiology and treatment of the major dementia diseases seen in humans (Colorado State University, n.d.). Knowing that neurodegenerative diseases arise from the toxicity and clumping of misfolded proteins (Tittelmeier et al., 2020), there is value in understanding how these protein aggregates arise and how they may be prevented or treated. Tittelmeier et al. (2020) goes on to explain how molecular chaperones are involved in the aggregation of these misfolded proteins byway of defective clearance mechanisms.

Chaperones monitor and prevent the misfolding and subsequent aggregation of proteins, making them important in the regulation of amyloid formation that could determine the progression of neurodegenerative diseases (Tittelmeier et al., 2020). Chaperones can detect misfolded proteins by recognizing the hydrophobic amino acid sequences located in the misfolded proteins that are not usually exhibited in their properly folded state (Tittelmeier et al., 2020). Evidently, chaperones are essential to the quality control of the proteome. The mechanisms of quality control associated with chaperons consists of regulating the folding of nearby proteins and the refolding of abnormal proteins so that they can display normal functioning states, while also destroying misfolded proteins with the ubiquitin-proteasome system (UPS) to prevent any further damage that could be incurred from aggregation (Tittelmeier et al., 2020). For example, several models reviewed by Tittelmeier et al. (2020) show that prion disease progression is increased when the concentration of the molecular chaperone Hsp 70 is decreased in the cytoplasm or endoplasmic reticulum. Although in most instances chaperones regulate correct protein folding to protect against misfolding and clustering and consequently prevent prion-like propagation, Tittelmeier et al. (2020) explores conflicting results where chaperons exacerbate the problem of protein misfolding and toxicity and thus failing to maintain protein homeostasis. Tittelmeier et al. (2020) states that protein aggregation can result from inadequate quality control of proteins when protein quality control machinery, such as chaperones, fail to maintain protein homeostasis. For example, when the Hsp 70 molecular chaperone tries to dissolve amyloid clusters, the rate of prion like propagation can increase due to the fragmentation of these aggregates leads to more toxic species that are more likely to spread and seed, unlike what is demonstrated when chaperones successfully dissolve protein aggregates that are not capable of seeding or propagation (Tittelmeier et al., 2020). This relationship between molecular chaperones and the propagation of prion-like proteins is significant because molecular chaperones can be further researched to uncover how they may be used to develop therapeutic agents to prevent the progression of neurodegenerative diseases. However, this may not be effective with increasing age since protein quality control network decreases and is less effective which allows neurodegenerative diseases to manifest themselves (Tittelmeier et al., 2020. As a result, understanding the contradictory roles of chaperones in interfering or further aggravating neurodegenerative progression is essential to develop effective therapies that can be used to treat such diseases.

Inheritance of Phenotypic Traits and Prions in Yeast Cells

Uncovering how and why proteins misfold can have positive implications for human and animal health issues. The misfolding of prions may arise spontaneously or with the chance of interaction of two or more non-prion molecules, both of which occur at higher protein concentrations (Derkatch et al., 2001). Since misfolded prions arise more when their respective host-encoded prion protein is overproduced, it is important to recognize factors that influence the spontaneous appearance of prions that may add to phenotype variability, such as those seen in yeasts. For example, Halfman et al. (2012) revealed that yeast cells expressing the Sup35 prion protein in its non-prion state can spontaneously switch to its misfolded prion state at a frequency of about 1 in 10^6. They state that the Sup35 prion is a translation-termination factor, where its misfolded prion form results in insoluble fibres, which causes a reduction in translation–termination activity by increasing stop codon read-through to generally translate more proteins; thus producing a variety of new phenotype traits. The seeding caused by the molecular chaperone Hsp104 in yeasts ensures inheritance of prion phenotypes by daughter cells (Halfmen et al, 2012). Phenotypes encoded by prion proteins can be inherited, which is supported by the fact the rates at which cells switch into and out of the prion state increases when cells are not well adapted to their environments and perhaps new phenotypes have a better chance of being beneficial for yeast survival (Halfmen et al, 2012). This increased rate of spontaneously prions switching into their misfolded prion state may be a direct consequence of the effects that diverse stress factors from the environment may have on protein folding and homeostasis (Halfmen et al, 2012). Similarly in mammals, multiple prion strains can self-propagate in the same host and exhibit distinct, heritable phenotypic traits (usually associated with disease processes), where these various strains from the same primary amino acid sequence may be as a result of structurally distinct misfolded prion shapes or conformations (Collinge & Clarke, 2007). Research done on the field of yeast prions have demonstrated a much wider biological importance of prion-like mechanisms, that may not lead to pathological processes, and have allowed direct confirmation (through experimentation of yeast cells) of the molecular mechanisms of prions that were previously hypothesized or proposed from work done with mammalian prions; however, mammalian prions are highly pathogenic and can vary from yeast prions (Collinge & Clarke, 2007). Understanding the reasoning for processes associated with protein misfolding and its resulting protein-based inheritance can have positive implications in the understanding of prion-like pathobiology, aging, and the evolution of cellular processes.

The unique ability of prions to misfold and propagate pathogenic information in the absence of genetic information can be useful to gain insight on neuro-degenerative disorders involving protein misfolding. The mechanism of prion propagation is also seen in other common neurodegenerative diseases, like Alzheimer's, that display prion-like propagation (Tittelmeier et al., 2020). As a result, researching prions can give insight on how to prevent and treat such diseases. The infectious characteristic of prions requires attention due to the fact that "within" and "cross-species" transmission is possible, such as the transmission of BSE from cattle to humans (Collinge & Clarke, 2007). As a result, new and potential prion pathogens have to be monitored, such as CWD from deer and elk, to prevent transmission to humans. Alongside this, further research needs to be conducted to determine the detailed structures of prions and their associated functions to reveal the exact mechanism of their propagation (Belay & Schonberger, 2005). This will help to learn how prions may express different phenotypic traits without genetic material, such as those seen in the differing disease phenotypes in mammals and the inherited phenotypes demonstrated in yeasts cells, to develop treatments and implement public health measures on how to prevent their propagation. All in all, further understanding of prions are required to determine how prions can refute fundamental biological principles by encoding phenotype information with amino acid sequences and learn about how prions propagate to fill in gaps in understanding about how neurodegenerative disorders with prion-like propagation arise and progress.

CHAPTER 4
Prions: Structure, Cellular Biology & Genetics

MEHVISH MASOOD

The Prnp Gene

Prions are formed through the misfolding of the prion protein (PrP), which is a protein that is encoded by the *Prnp* gene (Colby & Prusiner, 2011). The *Prnp* gene, which is located on chromosome 20 for humans("PRNP prion protein [Homo sapiens (human)] "), encodes the PrP protein open reading frame on one of its exons for all known species. This is despite having two to three exons present on the gene (Basler et al., 1986; Westaway et al., 1987; Hsiao et al., 1989; Gabriel et al., 1992). RNA seq analysis shows that the RNA of the *Prnp* gene is present all around the body and has its highest levels present in the brain ("PRNP prion protein [Homo sapiens (human)] "). Alignment of multiple translated sequences of the *PrP* gene shows a high degree of homology between the *Prnp* genes of mammalian species, which suggests that the PrP protein retention occurred due to an important purpose (Colby & Prusiner, 2011). However, the exact function of the gene is unknown with studies suggesting that the PrP protein has some function with protection of brain cells from injury, synaptic formation and the transportation of copper in cells ("PRNP gene", 2020).

The PrP Protein

Studies on Syrian hamsters show that the normal form of the PrP protein (PrP^c) is 254 residue protein that is post-translationally modified to make a 209 residue protein with two glycosylation sites and a GPI anchor. The first post translational modification removes an amino-terminal peptide sequence and the second is a carboxy-terminal peptide that directs the GPI anchor. The GPI anchor tethers the PrP protein as a lipid-linked anchor to the external cellular membrane (Colby & Prusiner, 2011). Also, modeling has shown that this protein is a four-helix protein that has four regions of secondary structure, denoted as H1, H2, H3 and H4 (Gasset, et al., 1992; Huang, et al., 1994). The form of PrP protein that induces disease (PrP^{Sc}) has no difference in terms of posttranslational modifications (Stahl et al., 1993). Thus it is also a 209 residue protein with a GPI anchor and has the same primary structure as PrP^{c}. Instead, PrP^{c} and PrP^{Sc} differ in terms of shape. PrP^{c} is rich in α-helical content and not in β-sheet content, while the inverse is applicable to PrP^{Sc} (Pan et al., 1993). The secondary protein structures of α-helices and β-sheets are caused by intramolecular hydrogen bonding within the amino acid backbone and have distinctive shapes: α-helices having a coiled up conformation and β-sheets having a pleated sheet conformation. Relative changes in the PrP^{c} and PrP^{Sc} shape cause a difference in protein hydrolysis: PrP^{c} is comparatively easier to digest by proteases under the same conditions. The limited hydrolysis of PrP^{Sc} often creates a shorter 142 residue polypeptide, which is denoted as PrP 27-30. Polymerization into amyloids can occur from PrP 27-30 in the presence of detergents and such polymers provide a useful means of detecting prions. However, such polymers are not essential in prion diseases and do not have to be present. Notably, not all forms of PrP^{Sc} are resistant to hydrolysis. These protease sensitive forms are referred to as sPrP^{Sc} (Colby & Prusiner, 2011).

The transition from PrP^{c} to PrP^{Sc}

The conversion of PrP^{c} to PrP^{Sc} is required for prion propagation. The mechanism of this transition has had several proposals. The first theory, the heterodimer model, proposes that the physical interaction between directly one PrP^{c} and one PrP^{Sc} causes the conversion. As in, the spontaneous transition of a single PrP^{c} to PrP^{Sc} is unlikely to occur due to the high energy barrier. As a result, the interaction between one PrP^{c} and one PrP^{Sc} catalyzes the change and forms a homodimer of PrP^{Sc}. This homodimer may dissociate following the conversion or aggregate to a PrP^{Sc} polymer. However, notably, this aggregation is a secondary process and so is not obligatory for the conversion to happen (Shkundina & Ter-Avanesyan, 2007). The polymerization model provides an alternative theory for the conversion of PrP^{c} to PrP^{Sc}. This model suggests that oligomerization is a necessary step in this conversion as opposed to a secondary process. The oligomerization of PrP^{Sc} is considered to be the rate determining step and is considered to be the intermediate in transformation. Under this theory, there are two variants in relation to oligomerization. The first variant suggests that PrP^{c} and PrP^{Sc} coexist in dynamic equilibrium and a shift towards PrP^{Sc} occurs for oligomers to form. The formation of an oligomer by PrP^{Sc} attachment causes PrP^{Sc} stabilization. If attachment does not occur, PrP^{Sc} will transition back to PrP^{c}. The other variant under the polymerization model suggest that the conversion occurs just before attachment to the oligomer (Shkundina & Ter-Avanesyan, 2007). However, in relation to the polymerization model, studies into transgenic organisms have shown how oligomerization isn't a necessary component for prion propagation. As in, transgenic Syrian hamsters were modified to express mouse PrP and Syrian hamster PrP. When the mouse prions replicated, plaques were not found and, when the hamster prions replicated, plaques were created. This thereby shows that plaques replication need not accompany replication (Prusiner et al., 1990). However, there is still evidence that supports the polymerization model (Caughey, Kocisko, Raymond, & Lansbury, 1995). Furthermore, it is important to discuss that, in addition to these models, conversion may require cofactors to aid with it. Notably, these cofactors have yet to be identified and so are often referred to as protein X. The binding of protein X to PrP^{c} is presumed to allow the interaction between PrP^{c} and PrP^{Sc}, and therefore enable the conversion to happen (Colby & Prusiner, 2011). Therefore, higher levels of protein X is hypothesized to increase prion-related disease, while lower levels of protein X could either reduce or even abolish such diseases.

The subcellular location of PrP^{c} to PrP^{Sc} conversion has been studied using various methods. One includes investigating prion-infection lines in scrapie-infected neuroblastoma cell lines (Colby & Prusiner, 2011). Within scarpie cell lines, conversion to PrP^{Sc} occurs after the PrP^{c} protein has been trafficked to the cellular membrane and anchored to the external cellular membrane through the use of a GPI anchor (Stahl et al., 1987; Borchelt et al., 1990; Caughey and Raymond, 1991). Following the movement to the cellular membrane, the PrP^{c} protein appears to re-enter the cells through subcellular compartments. These compartments are likely to be caveolae-like domains, which are cholesterol rich and detergent soluble membrane (Gorodinsky and Harris, 1995; Taraboulos et al., 1995; Vey et al., 1996; Kaneko et al., 1997; Naslavsky et al., 1997). At this point, the PrP^{c} protein may be converted to PrP^{Sc} or partially degraded (Taraboulos et al., 1995; Peters et al., 2003).

Incubation Times

Incubation times, which are defined as the shortest span of time between inoculation and time of disease, can vary. Incubation periods have shown to be short when the prion sequence introduced is identical to the host animal. As in, the prion sequence is from the same host animal. However, if a prion introduced is from a different species of the host animal, which would have a distinct prion sequence as well, the incubation period is prolonged. This varies substantially between separate animals and, for some inoculated animals, they don't develop prion related diseases (Carlson et al., 1989; Telling et al., 1994; Telling et al., 1995; Tateishi et al., 1996). The inability for some animals to not be able to develop prion related diseases when exposed to prions of other species is referred to as the species barrier.

Recognizing Prion Proteins

The ability to recognize proteins that have prion-like properties would be incredibly beneficial for prion-related research. In accordance to that, one study used *S. cerevisiae* prion proteins to find a criteria for prion identification. *S. cerevisiae* proteins are known to be rich in glutamine and asparagine residues. Also, PrP regions that were glutamine-rich tended to form amyloid fibrils *in vitro* (Perutz et al., 1994). So, it was hypothesized that regions rich with glutamine and asparagine, amino acids with highly similar properties, could be used to identify prion proteins. So, an analysis that checked for continuous segments of 30 glutamine and asparagine residues were searched for in the *S. cerevisiae* and *Drosophila melanogaster* genomes (Michelitsch & Weissman, 2000). This analysis showed that these continuous segments are fairly common and are encoded in many proteins of both genomes, which may suggest that prions are not rare in nature. However, not all prion-like proteins have contiguous glutamine and asparagine residues. Thus, this was not found to be a reliable method of being able to identify prion-like proteins. On the other hand, some research suggests that the presence of yeast prion determinants may cause specific cytoplasmically inherited phenotypes (Michelitsch & Weissman, 2000). With this being the case, research has been put into studying this.

Transgenic Organism Research

Transgenic mice that have altered expression of PrP have been studied to get insights into prion related disorders. Mice with knockout *Prnp* genes, which means that the *Prnp* gene has been removed from them, have been created. These mice were shown to be resistant to prion related diseases (Büeler et al., 1992; Büeler et al., 1993; Prusiner et al., 1993; Manson et al. 1994), which supports the need for the PrP protein for prion diseases. Notably, for some of these studies, altered synaptic behaviour was present when the gene was knocked out (Collinge et al., 1994; Whittington et al., 1995). In other studies, synaptic behaviour was not altered when with the knockout gene mice (Lledo et al. 1996). Other studies have looked to express various levels of wild type the *Prnp* genes in Syrian hamsters. Incubation times, which as mentioned before are the time between inoculation and clinical signs of the disease, were shown to be inversely proportional to the PrP expression (Prusiner et al., 1990). Transgenic mice have also had mutations introduced in the *Prnp* gene to study the impact of specific mutations. A mutation that has been introduced to the mouse PrP gene had a proline to leucine change on position 101. This mutation corresponds to the change that occurs in Gerst-mann-Sträussler-Scheinker disease (GSS). Neuropathological characteristics of prion diseases and accumulation of an abnormal isoform of PrP occurred in these mice (Hsiao et al., 1990; Tremblay et al., 2004).

Strain Variability

The ability for prion protein to acquire and induce different conformations is referred to as strain variability. This fundamental property of prion protein is determined by the primary amino acid sequence of Prp, which limits the amount of conformations it is able to make. The difference in strain viability changes the properties of prion related diseases. As in, it causes a variation in terms of incubation periods, clinical symptoms and even the ability to cross the species barrier (Shkundina & Ter-Avanesyan, 2007). The impact of different conforma-tional states was first found when laboratory hamsters were infected with two different strains of mink transmissible spongiform encephalopathies (TSEs). When comparing the two strains, they showed different incubation periods, clinical symptoms and the protein hydrolysis occurred in different regions (Bessen & Marsh, 1994). Alternatively, for Creutzfeldt–Jakob disease (CJD) several strains have been identified with varying phenotypes (Collinge et al., 1996).

Modes of Transmission

In accordance to the various prion diseases, the different structures and changes of the *Prnp* gene and Prp protein can cause a change in the transmissibility of the disease. For example, human prion diseases can either be genetic or trans-missible (Colby & Prusiner, 2011). Approximately 40 different mutations in the PrP gene have shown to cause heritable prion diseases. Germline mutations in the *Prnp* gene can cause prion diseases such as GSS or Fatal familial insomnia (FFI). Alternatively, somatic mutation or spontaneous conversion from PrPc to

PrPSc can cause Sporadic CJD. Transmission of prion disease can also occur through ritualistic cannibalism, as with Kuru disease, or through infection from contaminated medical equipment etc., as with Iatrogenic CJD. Notably, most forms of prion disease include neuropathological changes such as PrP deposition or vacuolation (Colby & Prusiner, 2011).

Prion related diseases do not only occur in humans, they can happen in other animals as well. Note that within humans prion diseases cause neuropathological changes such as PrP deposition, while within animals prion diseases occur as infectious disorders (Colby & Prusiner, 2011). Scrapie, a disease that has been documented for hundreds of years within sheep, is an infectious disease that does not seem to affect humans, mice and hamsters. Modifications in the PrP protein render some sheep more susceptible to scrapie and so selective breeding can be used to eradicate scarpie within sheep. Scarpie is also able to persist with the soil for years and is often used as a research tool due to its inability to impact humans, amongst other reasons (Colby & Prusiner, 2011). Bovine spongiform encephalopathy (BSE) or mad cow disease is a prion related disease that has caused massive epidemics for cows. In the 1970s, a change in the extraction method of meat and bone meal (MBM), a high-protein nutrient supplement for cows, caused cows to develop BSE. This led to many cows having to be slaughtered and a change in feeding habits to prevent this (Colby & Prusiner, 2011). Another prion related disease is chronic wasting disease (CWD), which has been reported in a variety of animals that mule deer, white-tailed deer and elk. CWD is an infectious disease that seems to be highly transmissible between different species of animals (Colby & Prusiner, 2011).

Expanding the Definition of Prions

Neurodegenerative diseases such as Alzheimer's and Parkinson's' disease are hypothesized to be prions as well. This is for several reasons. As mentioned before, Prp oligomerization is possible and it creates amyloid plaques. These amyloid plaques are thought to cause tissue damage and cell death, and are also present in other neurodegenerative diseases such as Alzheimer's and Parkinson's' disease (Colby & Prusiner, 2011; Prusiner, 1984). As these plaques are also found in neurodegenerative diseases, it can suggest that neurodegenerative disorders are due to prions as well. Furthermore, some studies using transgenic mice and cell cultures also support a prion-like, self-replicating mechanism for neurodegenerative diseases like Alzheimer's as well (Colby & Prusiner, 2011). Notably, for neurodegenerative disease to be prions, they must take up specific prion-like characteristics. This includes but is not limited to having β-rich structures that are toxic to cells, becoming less toxic when amyloid aggregation occurs, and mutations causing neurodegenerative disorders that facilitate the protein to a prion state (Colby & Prusiner, 2011). Further research and studies into neurodegenerative diseases are needed to confirm if prion designation or prion-like mechanisms are involved with them.

Conclusion

Prions have a unique type of structure, cell biology and genetics in association with them. Despite having the same primary sequence of the normal PrPc, PrPSc has a different structure that has an increased amount of beta sheets as opposed to alpha helices, which is a change that causes a diseased state for the protein. The transition occurs through the interaction of the two forms. However, the exact mechanism for the change has different but unconfirmed theories. Furthermore, research has looked into the impact of changing the *Prnp* gene and PrP expression to discover properties of prions. The impact of strain variability can change the course of prion-related diseases, which include properties like transmission. On the other hand, neurodegenerative diseases like Alzheimer's may be prions as well. With all this, more research needs to be done to get a more complete picture of prions as a whole and to look at the fascinating way that prions function.

CHAPTER 5
Human Prion Diseases: Causes, Symptoms & Diagnos
ISHPREET CHANA

Throughout the years, prion diseases (Prion is short for "proteinaceous infectious particle") have affected and caused death for many individuals. Prion diseases are rare neurological disorders that occur due to various reasons, such as mutations. A specific gene in the DNA code for the prion protein in the body is referred to as the PRNP gene. The prion protein synthesized is referred to as PrPc and is located on the surfaces of cells. Prion diseases occur after the PrP undergoes a misfolding in the protein folding process, and this variation is referred to as the prion (PrPSc). Alongside this, the prion protein can fold in various ways, giving rise to various strains of the prion. Moreover, polymorphism occurs at codon 129 which is also known as M129V in the PRNP gene, which forms different genotypes: 129 homozygous methionine (MM), 129 homozygous valine (VV), and 129 heterozygous methionine-valine (MV) (Karamujic et al., 2020). Through scientific research, led to different prion diseases to be developed such as: Creutzfeldt Jakob Disease (CJD), Gerstmann Straussler Scheinker (GSS), Fatal Familial Insomnia (FFI), variably protease sensitive prionopathy (VPSPr), and Kuru. The purpose of this article is to provide insight regarding the causes, symptoms, and the different types of diagnosage techniques of each prion disease.

Creutzfeldt-Jakob Disease (CJD)

The Creutzfeldt-Jakob Disease (CJD) is a rare class of neurological brain disorders in which the primary cause is changes within the prion protein (PrP). There are four classifications of CJD, which cause different symptoms and invoke different levels of severity. The different types include: sporadic, genetic, and acquired (Iatrogenic and Variant). The sporadic Creutzfeldt-Jakob Disease (sCJD) is the most common type of the CJD that occurs in approximately eighty five percent of the cases observed and it is a spontaneous process which can potentially arise from a random error found in a protein sequence (Prusiner, 1991). The genetic Creutzfeldt-Jakob Disease (gCJD) is an autosomal dominant inherited disease and a mutation is the predominant cause for the disease. gCJD can be inherited, if an individual has a family member that possesses the gene, or it can impact an individual without having any family history. According to a study, it was observed that it was inherited without having any family history impacting it, in almost fifty percent of the cases (Knight, Collins, 2000). The mutation is found in the PRNP gene and this further causes midfloding which leads to the production of PrPSc in the brain, through the abnormal synthesis of protein. Moreover, the mutation observed is a point mutation in the PRNP gene. For instance, insertions or deletions in the amino acid sequence of a polypeptide can generate point mutations in the PRNP gene. Within the acquired case, the prion is caused by various substances and this produces different forms of the CJD strain such as: iatrogenic, and variant. The prion in the iatrogenic CJD (iCJD), originated from humans or can arise from the duration of surgical procedures, such as blood transfusions. For example, it was found that high rates of iCJD developed from needles used for the treatment regarding the human growth hormone which was contaminated (Imran, Mahmood, 2011). Furthermore, the first ten cases of vCJD were discovered in 1996 within the United Kingdom. The variant CJD (vCJD) arises from Bovine Spongiform Encephalopathy (BSE) which is a disease that originates from cattle or from the contamination of food. BSE, commonly referred to as the "Mad Cow Disease", is a disease that is caused by the misfolding of prions and was discovered to arise amongst cattle and the version that humans may obtain is referred to as vCJD. Moreover, the codon 129 genotypes and the type of PrPSc impact the symptoms. For example, the 129 MM genotype led individuals to have more aggressive personality changes followed by rapid spread of dementia in vCJD. Furthermore, age does not have an impact when an individual is affected with the types of CJD. However, in most cases, it was found that sporadic CJD arose more commonly in middle aged adults and variant CJD arose more commonly in younger individuals (Knight, Collins, 2000). The symptoms of the types of CJD are relatively similar but follow some differences. For instance, individuals with sCJD experience symptoms that affect primarily the function of the central nervous system and the severity of the symptoms gets worse in the course of a couple of months. Whereas, patients with vCJD experience behavioural symptoms first while neurological symptoms develop later after a couple of months. ICJD does not have a definite path of which symptoms develop first as it depends on how an individual became exposed to the disease. For gCJD the development of the symptoms are the same as sCJD but it takes around two years for the symptoms to progress and worsen. For sCJD, gCJD, and iCJD, some of the early symptoms may include: mood swings, lack of interest in social aspects of life, memory loss, and the major symptom is dementia and myoclonia. After some weeks, an individual may potentially experience lack of muscle coordination, due to damage towards the cerebellum, which is known as cerebellar ataxia. The cerebellum is known as the part of the brain that is responsible for controlling movements. Symptoms that occur later include: blurred vision and speech, and this progressively leads to an individual losing all capability to do them, which is known as akinetic mutism and this eventually leads to death due to pneumonia. In a study it was found that, during four to five months after acquiring sCJD, the average human is approximately seventy percent dead and within a year an individual dies due to the rapid spreading of the disease. Moreover, the early symptoms for vCJD include severe depression, anxiety, insomnia, withdrawal from society and later symptoms are the same as sCJD, iCJD, and gCJD.

Gerstmann-Straussler Scheinker Syndrome

The Gerstmann Straussler Scheinker (GSS) is classified to be a transmissible spongiform encephalopathy (TSE) disease, also caused by a mutation in the PRNP gene. Through the mutation, the PrPSc undergoes a misfolding during the protein folding process and this causes many problems within the central nervous system. Some problems that arise in GSS are that the misfolded PrPSc is found within the brain complex, but primarily in the thalamus and cerebellum. After the misfolded PrPSc genes build up within the regions of the brain, they cause neurons to be destroyed, which further lead to various symptoms. The cause of this disease can be spontaneous and develop without any family history being present which is referred to as "de novo variant". This type of variant develops during pregnancy and specifically during the formation of the egg. Alongside this, this variant only affects the child and no other family member is affected. Moreover, it can also be an autosomal dominant, in which the carrier parent passes the gene to their offspring. According to scientists, there is a fifty percent chance that the carrier parent to pass the abnormal gene to their offspring, regardless of the sex. Furthermore, the symptoms vary depending on the type of mutation within the gene. For instance, in a study, a Japanese patient carrying the "P102L" mutation experienced leg hyperreflexia in the early stages as one of the symptoms (Imran, Mahmood, 2011). However, the symptoms are similar towards CJD. Early stage symptoms include: cerebellar ataxia, gait abnormalities, dysarthria, ocular dysmetria, dementia, ocular dysmetria, parkinsonia signs, areflexia, and spastic paraparesis. The later symptoms also involve the complete loss of muscle movement and speech, ultimately leading to a coma or death caused by pneumonia .

Fatal Familial Insomnia

Fatal Familial Insomnia (FFI) is considered to be an autosomal inherited disease, in which the PRNP gene undergoes a D178N mutation that is ultimately linked to the M129V polymorphism. FFI can also occur in either an inheritable manner where the abnormal variant can be inherited during the early stages of pregnancy, and not passed down by the affected parent. Furthermore, in some cases it was found that FFI developed without the mutation in the PRNP gene and it is known as sporadic fatal insomnia (SFI) (Imran, Mahmood, 2011). However, this circumstance is very rare to develop compared to FFI as the cause remains unknown. The severity and the duration of the symptoms vary depending on the 129 MM and 129 MV genotypes. The early symptoms include: insomnia, Myoclonus, dysarthria, seizures, dysphagia, and cognitive impairment. Over time the symptoms worsen and can lead to additional symptoms such as: excessive sweating, high blood pressure, rapid weight loss, delirium. According to studies, death usually occurs between six to thirty six months after acquiring FFI (2020).

Variably protease sensitive prionopathy

Variably protease sensitive prionopathy (VPSPr) is a sporadic prion disease as it occurs due to random mutations. VPSPr is also affected by the genotypes found on codon 129 in PrP. For example, individuals with the 129 MM genotype in the PRNP gene are protected against developing VPSPr compared to the 129 VV and 129MV genotypes (Imran, Mahmood, 2011). Furthermore, the symptoms and severity are impacted by the type of genotype. Generally, the symptoms are similar to the other types of prion disease, these include: ataxia, weight loss, depression, cognitive declinement, the loss of balance, and it eventually leads to death by pneumonia.

Kuru

Kuru was the first discovered prion disease known to mankind back in the 1920's. It first occurred within the Fore group in New Guinea where they would practice cannibalism with corpses during funerals and contracted this disease. The only potential causes of Kuru are consuming contaminated brain tissue or sores that are infected with kuru prions. The symptoms associated with Kuru occur in three stages. The first stage is where an individual with Kuru starts to lose some body control such as maintaining posture. The second stage is where the individual completely loses their capability to walk to perform daily activities. The third stage is where the individual is bedridden and tends to lose their ability to speak, which further causes malnutrition due to the inability to swallow. Death usually occurs within a year after contracting the disease due to the development of pneumonia.

Diagnosing

Diagnosing the types of prion diseases is a challenge since all the diseases form tiny holes in the tissue, caused by the TSE. To overcome these difficulties, many techniques are utilized in order to help distinguish between the various types of prion diseases. Moving on, there is no definite way of diagnosing any of the CJD cases as it is very difficult to diagnose and takes a while. However, the neurological images can provide distinguishing factors to help indicate what type of CJD an individual has. In the neurological tests for the acquired CJD, the images typically showcase amyloid plaques which are enclosed by spongiform lesions. In addition, individuals with the acquired CJD have higher amounts of PrPSc within the lymphoreticular system (Knight, Collins, 2000). Diagnosing sCJD and gCJD is extremely difficult, as it mimics other neurological disorders. However for sCJD and gCJD, standard neuropathological techniques are utilized to diagnose. One such technique is a biopsy, in which a small piece of the brain tissue is taken. However, there are limitations that arise due to this method, such as not removing a piece of the brain tissue from the infected area and performing surgeries toward the brain leads to risks and further complications. In addition, surgical tools pose a risk of spreading the disease if not cleaned properly, or destroyed after usage. Other tests used are: a blood test, to analyze for dementia, a computerized tomography (CT) scan to determine if there has been any strokes or tumors related to the brain, a magnetic resonance imaging (MRI), and an electroencephalogram (EEG), to determine if there has been any abnormalities in the brain, and a 14-3-3 protein test. The 14-3-3 protein test is a specific test that involves the spinal fluid. In this test a lumbar puncture is conducted, where a needle is inserted into an area below the spinal cord and a sample of cerebrospinal fluid is extracted and analyzed with the 14-3-3 protein. These techniques used alone cannot conclude that an individual has sCJD or gCJD, but they can play a supporting factor in the diagnosing process. To identify GSS, there are also clinical tests and imagery tests involved, along with the history of the patient. A molecular genetic test can be used to detect the abnormal variant in the PRPN gene. Additionally, various imaging techniques can be utilized to detect certain symptoms that arise within GSS. This includes: an EEG, a CT scan, a MRI, and a single photon emission computed tomography (SPECT). An EEG can be performed to measure the changes in the electrical activity within the brain and to detect seizures that may have occurred during the past. The CT scan is not as useful in the diagnosis for GSS but coupled with MRI it can help aid in the diagnosis process. For example, the CT can provide images regarding the cross-sectional regions for certain tissue structures, while the MRI can provide images regarding the cross-sectional for specific body tissues and organs. Therefore, these techniques used together can help conclude other conditions that mimic the GSS. However, MRI can be used alone, since it can provide images showcasing the abnormalities in the brain. SPECT is a type of CT scan that can be used by itself to help decode the diagnosis. In this technique, it is able to analyze how the blood flows towards tissues and organs through the use of a chemical tracer which is primarily radioactive material. Through this it can indicate areas of the brain that lack oxygen and nutrients due to the abnormal blood flow towards the blood vessels. Various techniques can be utilized to detect FFI and SFI such as: the 14-3-3 protein test, polysomnography, positron emission tomography (PET) scan, and the CT and MRI scans. The 14-3-3 test can be used in this case to analyze the evaluations levels of the cerebrospinal fluid. In some circumstances, no changes in the cerebrospinal fluid are observed. In these cases, the tau protein is examined in the cerebrospinal fluid. To aid in adding more clarity a new test called the real-time quaking induced conversion, is also used to detect for low levels of prions in the cerebrospinal fluid. Polysomnography is a sleep study that is used to analyze sleeping patterns within individuals. The PET scan produces three dimensional images that emphasize the metabolic activity within the brain and the decrease in the activity in the thalamus can help indicate the presence of FFI. The CT and MRI scan are utilized in the same coupled manner as in GSS. Moving on, for VPSPr the tests previously mentioned do not help diagnose the disease. However, in some cases the use of western blotting and analyzing for PrP immunochemistry have helped diagnose VPSPr. Western blotting is a technique that uses gel electrophoresis to separate the different proteins and in this case the PrP fragments with low molecular weight indicated towards VPSPr. The immunochemistry of the PrP showcased a patching distribution during the analysis, which helped indicate the presence of VPSPr. There are multiple methods utilized to detect Kuru. Kuru causes kuru plaques and spherical filaments to be formed, which aids in distinguishing the types of prion diseases. Additionally, it causes neuronal loss, and astrocytic microgliosis which is examined typically in grey matter. These techniques include: neurological exams and vision exams, an EEG, the 14-3-3 protein test, and blood tests. The TSE causes this disease to form tiny holes in the tissue which is examined through the microscope.

In conclusion, CJD has four different types of forms: sCJD, gCJD, iCJD, and vCJD. Each of these diseases has similar symptoms but the duration and the severity are impacted by the type of genotype at codon 129 in the PRNP gene. There are many techniques, both clinical and imagery diagnostic to help aid in determining the type of prion disease, but in some cases one technique works better than the other. Despite the fact that CJD, GSS, FFI, VPSPr, and Kuru are all different kinds of prion diseases, they all potentially lead to death. According to scientists there has not yet been a treatment to help an individual cure the disease. However, with advanced technology and ongoing research, one day scientists may discover a way to potentially help cure individuals that are affected by prion diseases.

CHAPTER 6
Biochemical Mechanisms of Prion Diseases

IVAN QUAN

To examine the biochemical mechanisms behind prion diseases, it is crucial to understand that a prion is a unique infectious agent in the form of a protein. All other known infectious agents such as viruses, bacteria, fungi, or parasites, use nucleic acids in the form of DNA or RNA to transmit their information from cell to cell and from organism to organism, generally composed of self-contained machinery allowing it to duplicate itself. In contrast, prions are proteins that transmit their information from protein to protein in the form of misfolding (Das & Zou, 2016). Proteins, composed of a long string of amino acids, will normally fold into a determined shape that allows them to carry out their function. Rarely however, proteins can misfold. While misfolding generally renders the protein to be inactive, in rare cases, misfolded proteins can result in abnormal protein activity, or can contribute to the progression of disease (Scheckel & Aguzzi, 2018).

In the case of prion diseases, the misfolded prion protein has several qualities that grant it the ability to become such a deadly infectious agent. The misfolded prion protein (PrPSc) will cause its normal protein variant (PrPC) to irreversibly misfold into PrPSc upon interaction (Priola, 2003). Additionally, misfolded prion proteins (PrPSc) will condense to form oligomers that can develop into amyloid plaque. As a PrPSc protein interacts with a normal variant PrP to convert it to PrPSc, these misfolded prion proteins will aggregate together. This protein aggregate can interact with and convert additional normal protein variants PrPC to PrPSc, which will continue to aggregate and build up the amyloid plaque (Rambaran & Serpell, 2008). Moreover, this prion aggregate is exceptionally stable. Not only will the individual proteins not revert to their normal folding pattern, but they are also resistant to mechanisms of protein destruction. This property allows amyloid aggregates to resist high heat, radiation, and proteases, enabling them to survive in the environment to infect another organism (Saunders et al., 2008). The amyloid aggregate created by the prion proteins is also resistant to biological protein destruction. Whereas the normal protein isoform is able to be digested by cellular proteases, the amyloid plaque is resistant to protease digestion, allowing the misfolded prion proteins to more easily accumulate within the body (Sajani & Requena, 2012).

With regards to prion diseases, it is this accumulation of PrPSc aggregates in tissue that results in the symptoms of disease. Accumulation of amyloid plaques within tissue will eventually lead to cell death (Brandner, 2003). Normal cellular PrPc protein is rich in alpha helices and is soluble in intracellular fluid. When interacting with PrPSc, PrPC will change its conformation to match PrPSc, becoming rich in beta sheets and becoming insoluble in intracellular fluid (Scheckel & Aguzzi, 2018). The misfolded prion protein is also able to spread between cells within tissue, meaning the problem is not necessarily localized to a single site in the tissue. Fragments of the misfolded protein oligomer may break off the large oligomer and migrate to surrounding cells to cause more proteins to become misfolded, growing the amyloid plaque once again (Rambaran & Serpell, 2008). As you might imagine, this process is a large positive feedback loop. As the amyloid plaque grows, more misfolded protein is available to convert cellular proteins to the misfolded form (Pöschel et al., 2003). Additionally, larger plaques are more likely to fragment and spread to surrounding cells in tissue, propagating the prion disease further within an organism. Overall, this results in the degeneration of tissue. Interestingly, this positive feedback loop is the reason that prion diseases are generally fatal shortly after the onset of symptoms (Imran & Mahmood, 2011). While the incubation period of prion diseases can last decades, the appearance of symptoms may indicate that the disease has already progressed to a point where the exponentially increasing PrPSc growth will rapidly propagate across tissue.

One group of prion diseases take the form of transmissible spongiform encephalopathies (TSEs). This disease affects the neural tissue of mammals such as sheep, cows, deer, and humans (Chesebro, 2003). The name of this disease originates from the sponge-like properties of neural tissue found in infected individuals. Normal neural tissue in the brain and nervous system is dense with neurons. However, images of tissue from individuals with transmissible spongiform encephalopathies display microscopic lesions across neural tissue, giving it a sponge-like appearance under a microscope (Atalay et al., 2015). These holes in the neural tissue were caused by misfolded prion proteins accumulating into oligomers, and causing cell death due to their neurotoxicity.

The mechanisms behind how PrPSc accumulation causes the neurodegeneration that characterizes TSEs is not very well understood. However, signs of apoptosis, a cellular mechanism promoting 'cell suicide', have been noted in infected animals (Brandner, 2003). PrPSc aggregates may place excessive oxidative stress on cells by inhibiting cellular antioxidant mechanisms, causing cells to become more susceptible to reactive oxygen species (Milhavet et al., 2000). The damage that reactive oxygen species causes to proteins, DNA, membranes, and other cellular structures may trigger the cell to initiate an apoptotic response, resulting in cell death, and in a broader view, damage to neural tissue. There has also been evidence for prion-mediated inflammatory events possibly causing cell death (Betmouni et al., 1996). In the central nervous system, microglia act as the resident macrophage cells, composing the main form of immune defence in the brain. In animals infected with TSEs, microglia can be seen surrounding PrPSc aggregates and consuming them (Prasad & Bondy, 2018). Although this could eventually degrade the protein aggregates, it could also enhance disease progression and spongiform degeneration in two ways. The now activated microglia secretes pro-inflammatory cytokines, prostaglandins, and nitric oxide to the site containing the amyloid plaques. In excess, this inflammatory response can produce levels of these molecules in toxic amounts to neural tissue (Prasad & Bondy, 2018). Additionally, as microglia are mobile cells, their movement could enhance the spread of PrPSc, thereby accelerating its propagation across tissue. Another mechanism behind the progression of neurodegeneration could be due to the PrPSc-mediated inhibition of PrPc (Aguzzi & Calella, 2009). As the prion disease progresses and the amount of PrPSc increases, PrPC function is correspondingly hindered, as it is converted to the misfolded isoform. PrPC is recognized as a cell surface glycoprotein present in all birds and mammals, and evidence suggests that PrPC binds copper ions to play a role in copper metabolism (Westergard et al., 2007). Since ionic copper is highly reactive, its coordinated uptake and transport is crucial to maintain proper neural tissue function. The structure of PrPC contains octapeptide repeats with high affinity for copper ions. The exact function of PrPC within copper metabolism however, remains unresolved. Researchers proposed that PrPC may be receptors for copper ion uptake, or may serve as a copper sink used to trap ionic copper, thereby regulating the intracellular copper concentration (Westergard et al., 2007). Nevertheless, the loss of PrPC function in later progression of TSEs may contribute to neuronal degeneration. Researchers have also proposed that the neurotoxicity associated with prion proteins may be the result of a toxic intermediate or by-product of the conversion from PrPC to PrPSc and large aggregate formation (Hughes & Halliday, 2017). The intermediate may exist in the form of smaller oligomers that compromise the integrity of the cell membrane, forming pores and forcing the membrane to become excessively permeable. Overall, while the exact biochemical mechanism behind the causes of neurodegeneration by prion diseases are not well understood, PrPSc formation and aggregation is known to contribute to the progression of disease.

Although neuronal death is understood to be the most apparent cause of neural deterioration and is the fatal outcome of prion disease, it is not the only way prions cause neurodegeneration. The first symptomatic effects of prion disease are caused by synaptic dysfunction (Senatore et al., 2013). In the early stages of prion disease, PrPSc is able to accumulate at neural synapses due to the high concentrations of PrPC normally present at synaptic structures. Prion disease has been linked to decreased expression of proteins involved in exocytosis and neurotransmission, suggesting that PrPSc accumulation interferes with synaptic transmission (Soto & Satani, 2012). Normally, nerves bind and release neurotransmitters at the synapse to communicate with adjacent nerves. Consequently, hindering the function of the synapse interferes with neurotransmission between nerves, causing the initial cognitive deterioration that accompanies TSEs. In addition to synaptic dysfunction, prions can cause dendritic degeneration in nerve cells in the early stages of TSE (Soto & Satani, 2012). Although the mechanism behind this process is unclear, it is known that PrPSc accumulation contributes to the increased expression of the Notch-1 intracellular domain (NICD) protein. NICD inhibits the growth of dendrites, which causes them to atrophy (Ishikura et al., 2005). A hallmark of dendritic atrophy can be seen in the reduction of branching displayed by neurons, which alters the connections made by the neuronal network. Ultimately, this leads to altered synaptic activity due to the reduction in connectivity, causing cognitive deterioration.

Creutzfeldt-Jakob Disease (CJD) is a TSE disease that affects humans, and three major forms of CJD exist: sporadic, familial, and acquired CJD (Mackenzie & Will, 2017). These forms are separated based on the mechanism of acquiring the disease. The mechanism behind the development of sporadic CJD is as its name implies, spontaneous and unpredictable. Rarely, a normal PrPC protein can spontaneously misfold into PrPSc, slowly convert other normal proteins into misfolded prion proteins, and eventually lead to sponge-like encephalopathy (Yegya-Raman et al., 2018). The onset of sporadic CJD can also arise genetically. Normally, the

PRNP gene encodes a PrPC protein. If this gene develops a spontaneous mutation in a somatic cell, it could lead to the gene encoding PrPC protein that is more susceptible to misfolding, or the mutated gene could encode a protein that will only fold into PrPSc (Yeyga-Raman et al., 2018). Either outcome will likely lead to the development of protein aggregates and the imminent neurodegeneration associated with TSEs.

Familial CJD, also known as inherited CJD, is a more rare form of the disease. Familial CJD is the result of an inherited mutation in the PRNP gene, such that it encodes a variation of PrPC that is more likely to misfold into PrPSc (Imran & Mahmood, 2011). Depending on the mutation that is inherited, individuals with mutated PRNP genes will have different likelihoods of developing CJD during their lifetime. While some mutations result in a near 100% probability of developing familial CJD, other mutations can result in a fraction of a percent chance to develop familial CJD (Clift et al., 2016). Mutations conferring familial CJD are gain of function mutations, being that the phenotype associated with the mutation is an outcome of the mutated gene, and not a loss of the functional gene. As a result, familial CJD is acquired dominantly, and requires only one copy of the mutant gene to possibly progress into disease (Chandra et al., 2019). Once the protein encoded by PRNP misfolds into PrPSc, its mechanistic progression towards disease is similar to that of sporadic CJD. Inherited mutations also form the basis of other human TSEs, including Gerstmann-Sträussler-Scheinker syndrome (GSS) and fatal familial insomnia (FFI), which, similarly to familial CJD, increase the likelihood of PrPC misfolding into PrPSc (Collins et al., 2001).

Rarer still is acquired CJD, which is the result of misfolded PrPSc being transmitted to an individual from an external source. Acquired CJD can be further divided into two categories: iatrogenic CJD, and variant CJD. The mechanism behind iatrogenic disease happens through contamination in medical treatment (Kobayashi et al., 2018). When conducting surgery in the brain or the head, the PrPSc protein isoform can enter a patient in multiple ways. Medical instruments used for surgery could be contaminated when used previously on an individual with CJD. Since prions are resilient to many common disinfection procedures, instruments used on someone with CJD could act as a fomite, transferring misfolded prion protein to the next patient (Saunders et al., 2008). Iatrogenic CJD can also arise from contaminated tissue transplant or fluid transfers. Historically, contaminated growth hormone, taken from individuals with undiagnosed CJD has been transmitted to individuals receiving growth hormone therapy (Kobayashi et al., 2018). Other procedures associated with transmission of PrPSc include

43

blood transfusions, corneal transplants, and dura mater grafts. In contrast, variant CJD did not originate in humans. The most well-known cases of variant CJD were transmitted from cows to humans via dietary consumption of beef infected with bovine spongiform encephalopathy (BSE) (Collee et al., 2006). Ingested prion proteins will be absorbed by the small intestine to be deposited into the lymphatic system. Microfold cells, present in the small intestine epithelium, are involved in a transcytosis process that intakes prions into microfold cells through membranous vesicles, depositing them on the basal side of the cell via exocytosis (Mabbott, 2012). It is hypothesized that migratory dendritic cells also play a role in the uptake of PrPSc protein, either by directly capturing it from within the intestinal lumen, or capturing PrPSc after it has crossed the intestinal epithelial layer through transcytosis. Eventually these dendritic cells may deliver the infectious protein to follicular dendritic cells, located within secondary lymphoid organs, including the spleen, lymph nodes, tonsils, and Peyer's patches (Collee et al., 2006). Within the secondary lymphoid organs, prion proteins begin to propagate inside maturing follicular dendritic cells. Since follicular dendritic cells express PrPC, this allows the ingested infectious PrPSc proteins to stockpile inside the lymphatic system (Mabott, 2012). After some accumulation of prion proteins has occurred, PrPSc is able to spread to the central nervous system through auto-nomic nerves. Researchers propose that PrPSc is able to spread between nerve cell synapses towards the central nervous system in multiple ways. When spreading in a stepwise manner, PrPSc may accumulate on the extracellular cell membrane face and convert the PrPC of adjacent nerve cells to PrPSc (Cobb & Surewicz, 2010). Transport can also occur through extracellular deposits, where plaques of PrPSc outside cells grow large enough to fragment and interact with adjacent nerves to propagate the prion protein towards the central nervous system. Spread could also arise directly through transport vesicles, where accumulation of PrPSc within the nerve cell leads to the creation of an extracellular vesicle that deposits PrPSc into neighboring nerve cells via endocytosis (Cobb & Surewicz, 2010). It is also hypothesized that PrPSc may be able to bypass the lymphatic system entirely, as evidence shows that PrPSc can be absorbed by the small intestine to be deposited directly into the bloodstream. Because PrPSc can freely cross the blood-brain barrier (BBB), it is able to infect the central nervous system through the blood (Urayama et al., 2016). Because PrPSc is present within the blood of an individual infected with variant CJD, this disease can spread via blood trans-fusions. If an individual with variant CJD donates blood, the prion disease has the ability to spread to the blood recipient by crossing the blood-brain barrier (Dietz et al., 2007). Regardless of the path it takes to get to the central nervous system, once PrPSc reaches the central nervous system, it is able to propagate to convert PrPC into the misfolded protein isoform to initiate the appearance of spongiform encephalopathy and subsequent neurodegeneration. Kuru is another form of TSE that can be transmitted through consumption of prion proteins. Kuru spread via the consumption of an infected human brain, in which PrPSc proteins would enter the digestive tract, making its way to the central nervous system through the blood or through the lymphatic system to autonomic nerves (Brandner et al., 2008).

Overall, although the precise mechanism by which prion diseases are initiated and propagated are not well understood, current knowledge on the topic nonetheless provides a solid interpretation on the broad view of the pathogenesis of TSEs. For TSEs to develop, PrPSc misfolded proteins must make their way into the central nervous system either by spontaneously misfolding in the brain, misfolding due to a genetic predisposition, or transport through lymphatic or circulatory systems. Once in the central nervous system, PrPSc is able to propagate by converting the normal cellular protein to the misfolded form, creating large misfolded aggregates. These aggregates begin the process of neurodegeneration first via synaptic degeneration and dendritic atrophy, further progressing into neuronal loss and spongiform encephalopathy in later stages of prion disease.

CHAPTER 7
Current and Emerging Therapeutic Approaches

SAPNA SINGH

Prion diseases are a group of rare and fatal neurodegenerative diseases that affect both humans and animals (Ludewigs et al., 2007). Human prion diseases are sporadic, genetic, and acquired with the most common disease deemed Creutzfeldt-Jakob Disease (CJD), having an annual worldwide death rate of approximately 1 person per million (World Health Organization [WHO], 2021). Prion diseases are caused by lethal agents called prions that induce abnormal folding of specific proteins known as prion proteins (Centers for Disease Control and Prevention [CDC], 2021). The accumulation of these abnormal proteins results in brain damage and rapid disease progression, however, further investigation on the nature and function of these proteins is warranted as it is still not completely understood (CDC, 2021).

Prion diseases, commonly known as transmissible spongiform encephalopathies (TSEs), are propagated by the conversion of normal forms of the prion protein PrPC, to the disease-causing isoform, PrPSc (Hwang et al., 2009). This conformational conversion can result in human prion diseases such as Creutzfeldt-Jakob Disease (CJD), Gerstmann-Straussler-Scheinker Syndrome, fatal familial insomnia, and Kuru as well as animal prion diseases including Bovine Spongiform Encephalopathy (BSE) in cattle, Chronic Wasting Disease (CWD) in deer, scrapie in sheep, and feline spongiform encephalopathy (CDC, 2021). Although decades of research have been invested into developing a cure for this disease, an efficient treatment is yet to be discovered due to the enigmatic nature of its pathogenesis. However, that being said, many alternative therapies have been cultivated to develop effective anti-TSE drugs (Ludewigs et al., 2007). Current therapeutic approaches for prion diseases include lentiviral and adeno-associated virus systems that target antibodies and siRNAs, anti-prion drugs that mainly target the prion protein PrPC and/or PrPSc, polycyclic drugs that prevent the conversion of PrPC to PrPSc, and many other treatments (Ludewigs et al., 2007). Over the years, there have been many clinical trials conducted for the treatment of prion diseases as well as constantly evolving, cutting-edge research that will hopefully lead to a breakthrough in discovering the cure for prion diseases in the near future.

The most predominant area of therapeutic research for prion diseases are drugs that are tested in three stages: *in vitro, in vivo,* and clinical studies. *In vitro* studies are manipulated to represent scrapie propagating cells whereas *in vivo* studies are used to represent scrapie-infected rodents (Ludewigs et al., 2007). Current drug therapies present successful results for both in vitro and *in vivo* trials however, the crucial challenge in developing an effective anti-prion drug is passing the clinical stages. Although most drugs prove to be effective in these preliminary stages, no drug has been observed to significantly prolong incubation times or increase survival in patients suffering from human prion diseases in clinical trials (Ludewigs et al., 2007). Additionally, because it is known that the disease stems from the conversion of PrPC to PrPSc, current drug strategies focus on directly inhibiting this conversion, degrading PrPSc isoforms, disrupting this process via accessory molecules, or altering PrPC expression and/or cell surface localization while keeping in mind effective strategies for penetrating the blood-brain barrier (Panegyres & Armari, 2013). As previously mentioned, many therapeutic approaches have been developed over the years against prion diseases, some of which are discussed in further detail in this chapter.

Anti-Infective Drugs

Polyanionic substances are highly abundant negatively charged macromolecules found in both the extracellular and intracellular environments that are accessible to many proteins for a variety of cellular processes (Urbinati & Rusnati, 2008). One such cellular function of polyanions is the ability to prevent TSEs and possibly disrupt the replication of prion diseases (Caughey & Raymond, 1993). Furthermore, a study conducted by Caughey and Raymond (1993) displays that sulphated polyanions can directly target infected cells like neurons and inhibit the accumulation of PrPSc. Thus, sulphated polyanions are a prime area of interest in the development of anti-infective prion drug therapies.

Dextran sulphate

The sulphated polyanion, dextran sulphate 500 (DS500) has been observed to be an effective drug against TSEs through *in vivo* mice studies. A single injection of this substance leads to reduced susceptibility to Scrapie and a prolonged incubation time in mice however, DS500 is also toxic to mice which poses a threat to its advancement to human clinical trials (Ludewigs et al., 2007).

Suramin

Suramin is another example of a polysulfonated drug that inhibits the production of the scrapie prion protein PrPSc by inducing misfolded PrPC in a post-endoplasmic reticulum/Golgi compartment (Ludewigs et al., 2007). This induced misfolding results in PrPC being redirected to acidic compartments, which prevent it from reaching cellular compartments where conversion occurs. Other derivatives of suramin have also been shown to inhibit *de novo* synthesis of PrPC and reduce the half-life of PrPC (Ludewigs et al., 2007).

Heparan mimetics

Heparan sulphate mimetics (HMs) are a class of polysulfated substances that play a role in viral infection by binding with heparin-binding proteins (Rusnati & Urbinati, 2009). HM2602 and HM5004 have been developed as possible drug therapies against multiple prion diseases as they block the PrPSc-37/67-kDa laminin receptor (LRP/LR)-HSPG binding while also inhibiting the absorption of the fatal PrPSc isoform into cells (Ludewigs et al., 2007). However, further drug development is warranted as only HM2602 was found to increase survival in scrapie-infected hamsters

Polyene antibiotics

Polyene antibiotics like amphotericin B (AmB) and MS 8209 are antifungal substances that have been shown to exhibit anti-prion properties in scrapie-infected hamsters (Ludewigs et al., 2007). These antibiotics seem to not only delay disease progression but also inhibit toxic PrPSc accumulation. In fact, studies using BSE and scrapie-infected murine models have reported increased survival times and delayed PrPres and glial fibrillary acidic protein accumulation (Ludewigs et al., 2007). Moreover, these antifungal agents may interact with cholesterol on the surface of cell membranes to impede the absorption of PrPSc into target cells, inhibit the replication of the scrapie agent to the peripheral nervous system, or prevent the conversion of PrPC to PrP^{Sc} (Ludewigs et al., 2007).

Designer peptides

Recent advances in ligand technology have allowed for the development of designer peptides that act as therapeutic agents for various diseases. Now, peptides can be intricately designed to exhibit similar affinities akin to antibodies and greater specificities compared to other small molecules and some antibodies (Shrivastava et al., 2009). In regards to prion diseases, scientists have developed β-sheet breaker peptides that decrease the susceptibility to prion diseases by disrupting the conformational structure of PrP (Ludewigs et al., 2007). More specifically, a 13-residue β-sheet breaker peptide (iPrP13), was found to reverse the structural conversion of PrPSc into a structure similar to PrP^C in a hamster ovary cell culture assay (Soto et al., 2000). Furthermore, *in vivo* studies that incubated scrapies with iPrP13 prior to injection reported a 90 to 95% decrease in the infectivity of PrPSc material and delayed appearance of clinical symptoms in mice (Ludewigs et al., 2007). Further development and analyses of these peptides may improve our understanding of the pathogenic conformational changes that occur in PrP and may provide an effective therapeutic approach to human prion diseases.

Tyrosine kinase inhibitors

Tyrosine kinase inhibitors (TKIs) are pharmaceutical drugs that interrupt the signal transduction cascades of tyrosine kinases enzymes. Tyrosine kinases are responsible for the activation of specific proteins through the mediation of cellular pathways. TKIs operate by blocking the phosphorylation of tyrosine kinases, a crucial step needed for the activation of these proteins (Thomsan et al., 2021). It is believed that tyrosine kinases play a role in the signal transduction pathway necessary for the conversion of PrP^C to PrPSc. Through a series of screening trials, it was found that the tyrosine kinase inhibitor STI571, is effective at arresting PrPSc production in prion-infected cells without disrupting the biogenesis, localization, or biochemical features of PrPC. STI571 also activated the lysosomal degradation of PrPSc and decreased its half-life from approximately 24 hours or more, to less than 9 hours (Ertmer et al., 2004). Tyrosine kinase inhibitors may act as a powerful tool in understanding the signalling pathways behind the conversion of PrP^C into its pathogenic isoform and can be further developed as an anti-prion drug.

Antiprion Antibodies

The field of immunotherapy has been widely investigated in the realm of prion diseases as antibodies are one of the fastest-growing agents of human therapeutics. Antiprion antibodies are synthesized against common peptide residues on the structural domain of PrP. One such common residue is the tyrosine-tyrosine-arginine repeat motif that contains a common tyrosine pair conserved across mouse, hamster, sheep, bovine and human PrP (Paramithiotis et al., 2003). Antibodies directed against this sequence repeat can recognize the pathological isoform of PrP and may unveil key information regarding the structure of PrPSc that remains somewhat ambiguous due to the limitations of low-resolution fragmentary structures that are currently available (Paramithiotis et al., 2003). Furthermore, studies have shown that antibodies directed against PrP^C can eradicate scrapie-infected cells containing PrPSc *in vitro* and prevent the progression of scrapies in transgenic mice models *in vivo* (Paramithiotis et al., 2003). Research using prion-knockout mice report successful production of anti-PrP antibodies however, further immunotherapy development is required as it is still unclear which PrP epitope (antibody-binding region)is the most effective target to disrupt prion propagation (Ludewigs et al., 2007). Additionally, autoimmune recognition of PrPC may induce unwarranted activation of signalling cascades, immunosuppression, and complement-dependent cellular lysis (Paramithiotis et al., 2003).

Monoclonal antibodies
The monoclonal antibody 15B3 was developed to specifically target PrPSc isoforms and is able to differentiate between benign PrP^C and the disease-associated form PrPBSE (Ludewigs et al., 2007). Antibodies synthesized against the C-terminal domain of PrP such as 6H4 and the antigen binding fragment Fab D18/D13, have been implied to block the binding domains of PrP^C and PrPSc as they inhibit the accumulation of PrPSc in neuroblastoma cells. More compellingly, when N2a cells are exposed to antibody 6H4, they are protected from scrapie infections, suggesting a potential cure for the disease (Ludewigs et al., 2007). Other monoclonal antibodies have also been found to inhibit prion replication and the development of prion diseases. White and colleagues (2003) investigated the effects of ICSM 35, an immunoglobulin-γ2b (IgG2b) monoclonal antibody developed against β-PrP conformations and ICSM 18 raised against α-PrP conformations on PrPSc accumulation. Using scrapies-infected mice, it was found that weekly injections of ICSM antibodies resulted in notable decreases of PrPSc concentrations in the spleen through Western blot analysis. Additionally, scrapies-infected mice that received a continuous treatment of ICSMs remained healthy for over 300 days compared to equivalent untreated mice that developed the disease (White et al., 2003). ICSMs provide sound evidence for the use of immunotherapy in combating prion diseases however, further development is

needed as the passive immunotransfer of anti-PrP antibodies shows no effect in the late incubation period when clinical signs are already developed (Ludewigs et al., 2007).

Combined antibodies

Some areas of research advocate for the use of combined antibodies in cell culture like the use of SAF34 antibodies that are directed against the octapeptide repeat residue, and SAF61 antibodies which when combined, inhibit PrPSc synthesis (Ludewigs et al., 2007). The advantage of employing a combined antibody approach is that multiple binding sites on the prion proteins can be inhibited which may result in an increased inhibition effect. For example, the epitopes for SAF34 and SAF61 are located on two different binding sites on the PrP for the 37/67-kDa LRP/LR protein which may disrupt the PrP-LRP/LR interaction and therefore, lead to the degradation of PrPC (Ludewigs et al., 2007). The 37/67-kDa LRP/LR protein which binds lamin-1 and prion proteins was found to be a receptor for both PrPC and the disease-causing isoform PrPSc, thus antibodies blocking the LRP-PrP interaction may inhibit PrPSc production as was seen with SAF34 and SAF61. Expanding on this, the polyclonal anti-LRP/LR antibody W3, was reported to arrest PrPSc propagation in scrapie-infected N2a cells and prolong survival in infected rodents (Ludewigs et al., 2007).

More recently, immunization and vaccination trials have been put forward as it is known that the immune response can antagonize the disease. As previously discussed, White and colleagues (2003) investigated the effects of passive anti-PrP immunization on scrapies through the use of two different monoclonal antibodies. However, the protective effects of passive immunization were only observed following intraperitoneal infection (White et al., 2003). Other studies have examined the effects of a single dose of 500 μg antibody injections on fatal PrP accumulation following exposure to scrapies. It was found that two different monoclonal antibody binding residues (34-52 of PrPC and 175-185 of PrPSc) prolonged the onset of clinical symptoms by approximately 20 days compared to other antibody binding PrP residues that exhibited a lower affinity (Buchholz et al., 2006). It is seen that passive immunity can prolong the survival of scrapie-infected animals and can restrict scrapie development after peripheral prion infection however, is challenged by the ability to maintain protective anti-PrP antibody levels (Buchholz et al., 2006).

Naturally, as passive immunity was investigated, advancements to develop active immunization against prion diseases have been studied. Research in this area mainly focuses on developing PrP-specific T-cell tolerance that is speculated to play a crucial role in preventing PrP-related autoimmunity (Buchholz et al., 2006). PrP-specific peptides or bacterially expressed recombinant PrP, in combination with various adjuvants, are employed in these trials. One study examined the immunization of wild-type mice using a polypeptide equivalent to helix-1 of human PrP where the human prion protein was indeed detected in an ELISA (Buchholz et al., 2006). Several other studies investigating active immunity have been conducted over the years, however, common to all studies is the finding that PrP-specific antibody responses are relatively low and in wild-type mice were never directed against PrPC (Buchholz et al., 2006). Although active immunization against prion diseases remains in its infancy, continuous advancements in research may unveil a breakthrough in this type of immunotherapy.

Anti-prion drugs: Symptomatic treatment

Many patients suffering from CJD exhibit a wide range of symptoms which poses a challenge to diagnosing the disease and providing effective treatment. Most patients report psychiatric symptoms such as depression, anxiety, psychosis, and hallucinations thus, anxiolytic and antipsychotic drugs like benzodiazepines are routinely prescribed to alleviate some of the symptoms (Ludewigs et al., 2007). Other drugs such as clonazepam and valproate are used as additional symptomatic therapy options for CJD-typical myoclonus. Additionally, case reports have indicated that some analgesic, antidepressant, antipsychotic, antimicrobial, and anticoagulant drugs may have the potential as an anti-prion drug (Ludewigs et al., 2007).

Pentosan polysulfate (PPS), a polyglycoside molecule, has been observed to affect PrP production, replication, and cell toxicity *in vitro* and thus, has the potential of being a prophylactic drug against prion diseases (Ludewigs et al., 2007). PPS is believed to compete with endogenous heparin sulphate proteoglycans as a coreceptor for PrP on its cellular surface however, cannot penetrate the blood-brain barrier following oral or parenteral administration (Burchell & Panegyres, 2016). Studies have shown that injections of PPS into the cerebral ventricles of mice following prion infection correlated with increased survival times in all cases (Burchell & Panegyres, 2016). In human case studies, treatment with PPS for CJD patients is limited however, some information on previous reports is available. In one case study, a 22-year-old male suffering from vCJD was treated with continuous intraventricular PPS (32 µg/kg/d) 19 months after the onset of clinical symptoms for a total of 31 months. This suggests that PPS is not only a safe and well-received therapeutic but also can prolong the life expectancy of patients (Burchell & Panegyres, 2016). Furthermore, an observational study in the UK investigated the effects of continuous intraventricular administration of PPS in seven patients with human prion diseases across a 6-month timeline. It was found that PPS was well tolerated over a wide dose range of 11-110 μg/kg/day and patient assessments reported one patient who remained stable, two exhibiting minimal deterioration in symptoms, and a significant clinical progression in one patient at the end of the study. This observational study provides convincing evidence for the use of PPS as an anti-prion therapy as the mean survival of all treated patients was greater than that of untreated patients that were reported through historical records (Bone et al., 2008). Due to the current limited number of observational trials, dose ranges of PPS vary widely, therefore, the next step in PPS therapy is to establish a safe and effective dosage that can be standardized to all patients (Burchell & Panegyres, 2016).

Future Prospects

Thus far, treatment for prion diseases is still in its discovery stages however, as seen, numerous alternative therapeutics have been developed in attempts to alleviate the daunting symptoms of the disease. Both passive and active immunotherapies have been investigated however, both strategies display differential levels of success in murine models. Furthermore, the advancement of active immunization therapies to human trials presents some challenges due to concerning side effects such as autoimmune meningoencephalitis (Burchell & Panegyres, 2016). Thus, although no effective cure has been created yet, researchers are focused on developing possible passive immunization strategies to target the disease's pathology in the near future. Coupled with this is the search for strategies that improve the earlier diagnosis of prion diseases as this would ensure timely treatment of passive immunization and would increase the chances of delaying disease progression and prolonging lifespan (Burchell & Panegyres, 2016). Such strategies may include the identification of prion disease biomarkers, predictive genetic testing and other screening tests (Panegyres & Armari, 2013). Moving forward, passive immunization could be targeted to at-risk populations such as those with known mutations in the PRNP gene, and can then progressively expand to whole populations or those with an increased risk of exposure (Burchell & Panegyres, 2016). In regards to vaccines, prion peptides provide a promising method for establishing possible CWD vaccines however, this would only be developed in the decades to come owing to the limited number of cases and lengthy process of human clinical trials (Ludewigs et al., 2007). Lastly, siRNAs may also be an effective approach to prion therapy as it could be directed against PRNP mRNA, LRP mRNA, and various other mRNAs that are essential for the life cycle of prions (Ludewigs et al., 2007). All in all, a better understanding of the cellular mechanisms involved in the conversion of PrP would allow researchers to develop specific treatments for prion diseases, and eventually, an effective cure.

CHAPTER 8
Epidemiology & Risk Factors of Human Prion Diseases
IVY QUAN

The purpose of epidemiology is to identify the etiology, risk factors, extent, history, and prognosis of a disease to inform the development of therapies and public health policies. Since the investigation into Scrapie, the first recorded prion disease, in 1732 (Zabel & Reid, 2015), epidemiological studies exploring the origin, transmission, and distribution of human prion diseases have assisted our current understanding of why and how these diseases occur. Human prion diseases have a variety of aetiologies: sporadic, familial, and acquired. They can originate sporadically by a randomly misfolded PrP protein, or via genetically inherited protein mutations. They can also be acquired through exposure to infected brain matter during a medical procedure, or ingesting infected food products, but cannot be transmitted through casual contact (Pederson & Smith, 2002).

A prominent example of acquired human prion disease is the Kuru epidemic that occurred amongst the Fore people of Papua New Guinea first documented in 1957 by Gajdusek and Zigas. Kuru means to shake or tremble, which was one of the main presentations of the disease alongside bouts of spontaneous laughter. Between 1957 and 1982, more than 2500 Kuru fatalities were reported: 67% of the fatalities were adult women, 10% were adult men, and 23% were children and adolescents (Pedersen & Smith, 2002). On average, the incidence of Kuru was 1%, but it was as high as 10% in some villages in the late 1950s. In 1959, researcher J.H. Bennett and his team proposed that Kuru was a genetic disease based on pedigree trees they tracked for Kuru cases. His study hypothesized that the Kuru disease was controlled by a single autosomal dominant allele where only homozygous dominant males of some allele K would demonstrate clinical presentations associated with Kuru. While homozygous dominant females are early-onset cases, and heterozygous females are late onset cases. The theory that only heterozygous females and not males displayed symptoms of clinically significant Kuru was to account for the fact that it seemed to disproportionately affect women (Bennett et al., 1959). However, there were no recorded cases of children being born with Kuru since 1959, and ages of disease onset gradually increased since the arrival of government officials and missionaries in the 1950s (Liberski et al., 2019). These observations seem to challenge Bennett's genetic hypothesis.

Along with the arrival of missionaries and officials to South Fore in the 1950s, the practice of ritualistic endocannibalism ceased. Additionally, the absence of reported Kuru cases in children born after 1954 suggests that the transmission of the disease to children stopped synchronously with the cessation of cannibalistic practices (Liberski et al., 2019). These observations point to the ingestion of infected flesh to be the main route of transmission for Kuru. The Fore people practiced funerary cannibalism, in which they would consume deceased kinsmen to mourn their passing. As per tradition, women were responsible for preparing the flesh and organs, including the brain, of their deceased kinsmen. Young children were also active in the ritual, but adult men were not as active and rarely ate the brain matter of dead women (Pederson & Smith, 2002). Looking at their traditions provides an explanation for why Kuru disproportionately affect adult women and children. Matthews, Glasse, and Lindenbaum (1968) were the first to propose that Kuru was transmitted through cannibalism. And they correctly predicted that Kuru would disappear in the next few decades given the absence of endocannibalism. It is now thought that the first case of Kuru was caused sporadically by a random misfolded protein, then consumption of that patient's infected brain matter allowed Kuru to spread throughout the Fore villages. Although the causative agent for Kuru was not yet discovered to be a prion protein, the Kuru epidemic led to early observations of supporting evidence for the prion hypothesis. Determination of the route of transmission also led to the estimation of the incubation period, or the time between infection and clinical onset of symptoms, of approximately 12 years (Alpers, 2008).

Moreover, modern genetics tests have determined there is no genetic basis for Kuru transmission. But, more recent genotyping studies have demonstrated that genetics can modulate an individual's susceptibility to the disease. According to Mead et al. (2008), heterozygosity at the codon 129 of the prion protein gene (PRNP) correlated with resistance to CJD, and heterozygosity was overrepresented in survivors of the Kuru epidemic. Homozygosity at codon 129 of PRNP, particularly two alleles coding for the amino acid methionine correlated with high susceptibility. Within a sample of 48 cases of Kuru in children and adolescents, approximately half were found to be homozygous for methionine at codon 129 (Mead et al., 2008). This suggests that methionine homozygosity increases an individual's susceptibility to Kuru and results in early onset cases. Discoveries of both the transmission route and risk factors for Kuru were instrumental in the epidemiological study of the bovine spongiform encephalopathy (BSE) epidemic in the 1980s.

BSE, or more commonly known as mad cow disease, is a form of TSE that originated in cows. The BSE and subsequent variant CJD (vCJD) outbreak in the United Kingdom during the 1980s and 1990s is another example of acquired CJD transmitted via consumption of infective tissues. It is also a clear demonstration of how etiological studies can inform public policies. Although the origin of the first case of BSE is unknown, there are several hypotheses. One theory is that the UK was among the first countries to begin feeding young cattle meat-and-bone meal (MBM), a high protein supplement containing mainly sheep and cow deemed unfit for human consumption. Young cattle demonstrate higher susceptibility to BSE, and this exposure may have led to the first cases recorded in the UK (Smith & Bradley, 2003). Another possibility is that cows supplemented with MBM were exposed to an infective agent that originated from scrapie (a TSE found in sheep). And yet another theory is that the first cases were sporadic protein folding mistakes that then spread to other cattle through the MBM ruminant feed chain (Smith & Bradley, 2003). The first case of BSE in cattle was discovered in 1986 when two cows displayed progressive neurological symptoms similar to scrapie. These first documented cases led to the development of clinically significant BSE in over 180,000 cattle in the UK (Smith & Bradley, 2003). Additionally, 1-3 million cattle may have been infected with the BSE agent but slaughtered for human consumption prior to displaying symptoms (Donnelly et al., 2002). The practice of feeding MBM to cattle was a vehicle for BSE because it was common practice for fallen stock and butcher's waste to be processed into MBM. So, cows ingesting the infectious components of another cow with BSE such as the brain, spinal cord, and retina, were at risk of being infected with BSE themselves (Smith & Bradley, 2003).

The BSE epidemic, its origins, and its mode of transmission is crucial to understand because it resulted in a public health crisis in which 10 atypical cases of CJD were reported in the UK during 1996 (Smith & Bradley, 2003). These cases varied from prior CJD cases because they were all early onset cases with more than half dying before the age of 40 (Pedersen & Smith, 2002). They were classified as variant CJD (vCJD), and there is strong epidemiological evidence for a causal relationship between a BSE agent and onset of vCJD. There are no confirmed vCJD cases in geographic areas without cases of BSE. Furthermore, the time between the exposure to cattle products containing BSE in 1984-1986 and the onset of the first vCJD cases in 1996 supports the unusually long incubation period previously noted for CJD (Pederson & Smith 2002). Although the exact mechanism for transmission is not clear, vCJD has been confirmed to be caused by ingestion of a cattle product containing BSE. Interestingly, although an estimate of 0.5 million BSE-infected cows were processed for human consumption (Pederson & Smith, 2002), there have been only 229 confirmed vCJD cases to date worldwide with a majority of cases identified in the UK (Surveillance for vCJD, 2019). This suggests the possibility of an inter-species barrier, and the inefficiency of the oral route of transmission across species. Genetic factors also undoubtedly play a role in vCJD transmission as a large majority of reported vCJD cases are homozygous for methionine at codon 129 of the PRNP. All UK cases apart from one, displayed methionine homozygosity (Saba & Booth, 2013). This is the same polymorphism that resulted in early onset and shorter incubation times for Kuru. Yet, it is still unclear if homozygosity for methionine increases susceptibility, shortens the incubation time, or both. Another contributor to the under predicted case numbers could be the public health measures placed to prevent the transmission of BSE amongst cattle and from cattle to humans.

In response to the identification of the MBM ruminant feed chain as the perpetuator of the BSE epidemic, ruminant feeding was banned for cattle in the UK in 1988. By 1992, new cases of BSE decreased by 40%, the delay being reflective of the 5-year incubation period for BSE (Smith & Bradley, 2003). However, this 1988 ban was not completely effective as there continued to be BSE cases born after the ban in areas with a high concentration of pig farms. This may be the result of cross-contamination, as ruminant feeding was not banned for pigs or chickens (Smith & Bradley, 2003). Therefore, after the emergence of the first cases of vCJD, the ruminant feeding ban was extended to include all farm animals that same year. A few years prior, in 1989, the UK also issued the Specified Bovine Offal (SBO) ban which banned bovine brain, spinal cord, tonsil, thymus, spleen, and intestines from the human food chain (Smith & Bradley, 2003). While the ruminant feed ban focused on controlling the transmission of BSE between cattle, the SBO ban targeted BSE transmission to humans, and is considered the most important measure to protect humans from consumption of BSE infected products. To further human protection the UK introduced the over 30-month (OTM) scheme in 1996 that relegated all meat from cattle over 30-months old to have bones, nervous tissue, and lymphatic tissue removed. Additionally, this regulation banned the consumption of British cattle over 30-months old (Smith & Bradley, 2003). The OTM rule was annulled in 2005 alongside a ban on the human consumption of cattle born before August 1996. Understanding the risks and etiology of BSE and vCJD informed public health decisions and policies which ultimately served to protect people from acquiring these harmful prion diseases. However, a less preventable form of CJD is sporadic CJD.

The origins for both Kuru and the BSE epidemic have been hypothesized to be a sporadic case of a prion disease. In fact, sporadic misfolding of the prion protein is the most common form of CJD and accounts for about 85% of all recorded cases with a mean age of onset at around 65 years (Pederson & Smith, 2002). There has been no evidence of clustering sporadic CJD cases, which suggests that casual and sexual contact are not viable transmission routes. These cases occur worldwide at roughly 1-1.5 cases per million per year across all age groups, while risk increases with age (Occurrence and Transmission, 2021). CJD incidence amongst the 65-74 year old age group was recorded in 2002 to be 3 per million per year, while the incidence in those less than 40 years old was 0.2 per million per year (Pederson & Smith, 2002). Therefore, in more recent years, the increasing trends of CJD incidence may be attributable to the world's ageing population. In fact, Japan recorded a CJD incidence of over 4.5 per million in 2014, which could be explained by Japan's hyper-ageing society (Nishimura et al., 2020). Age is thought to play a role in CJD onset because errors in cellular machinery are more likely to occur as we age. Similarly to Kuru and vCJD, another risk factor is the homozygous methionine polymorphism of codon 129 on the PRNP. 85% of sporadic CJD cases were genotyped as homozygous at codon 129 compared to 50% of the general population in Europe, and two thirds of the homozygous genotype displayed methionine homozygosity (Pederson & Smith, 2002). While the mechanism for the effect of codon 129 homozygosity on CJD is still unknown, it's consistency as a risk factor across all forms of human prion diseases is something to note.

Other inherited genetic mutations can also lead to the development of CJD, giving rise to familial cases. These differ from codon 129 polymorphism because they are controlled by an autosomal dominant mutation of the PRNP and have been identified as causative mutations. Single amino acid substitutions that lead to familial CJD largely occur near alpha-helical regions of prion proteins. They are thought to destabilize the alpha helix to facilitate its conformational change to a beta-pleated sheet, which is the molecular basis for the misfolding of a prion protein (Pederson & Smith, 2002). For example, a substitution replacing proline with leucine at codon 102 leads to a subtype of familial CJD called Gerstmann-Straussler-Scheinker (GSS) Syndrome. GSS differs from sporadic CJD in that it has an earlier onset averaging 48 years old, and a longer disease duration that averages 5 years (Pederson & Smith, 2002). Patients with GSS have a variety of clinical presentations, but most display cerebellar ataxia with amyloid plaques in the brain (Hsiao et al., 1989). Another substitution mutation found at codon 200 was found in more than 60 families of Libyan Jewish descent. Amongst those with this genetic mutation, the incidence of CJD is 100 times higher than the worldwide incidence (Meiner et al., 1997). Penetrance is the percentage of people with a particular genotype that expresses a phenotype; in this case, the percentage of people with the mutation who develop familial CJD. The penetrance for the causative mutation at codon 200 is 0.45 at 60 years old, and 1.0 in those over 80 years old (Meiner et al., 1997). The final well documented substitution mutation occurs at codon 178, and can be found in Finland, Europe, and Asia. This causative mutation is unique because it is modified by the codon 129 polymorphism. If the substitution occurs on the same allele as codon 129 coding valine, the resulting CJD is similar to sporadic CJD but with an earlier onset at around 46 years old and longer disease duration of 2 years (Pederson & Smith, 2002). However, if the substitution occurs on the same allele as a codon 129 for methionine, this results in a subtype of familial CJD known as familial fatal insomnia (FFI). FFI has a unique presentation which consists of early onset sensory and motor complaints in conjunction with severe insomnia. Patients with FFI have been found to have neuronal loss specifically within the thalamic nuclei responsible for relaying sensory information (Pederson & Smith, 2002). As more suspected CJD cases are genotyped, we can further our understanding of the etiology and distribution of familial CJD cases which may then assist diagnosis and early interventions.

Epidemiological studies of the acquired, sporadic, and familial CJD cases can inform the development of diagnostic and therapeutic tools as well as public health policies. Tracking CJD incidence and dispersion can help to identify risk factors such as age, or residence in the UK. Additionally, through tracking, it is clear that human prion diseases are rare and cannot be transmitted through causal or sexual contact. Transmission of TSEs only occurs when infected tissue containing an infectious prion protein enters an individual's blood stream via ingestion of the tissue or an abrasion. Within these acquired cases, and also for sporadic CJD, common risk factors include age and methionine homozygosity at codon 129 of PRNP. As demonstrated in the BSE epidemic, knowledge about these transmission routes and risk factors can aid the creation of guidelines and policies that protect people from acquired CJD which poses many challenges for public health.

CHAPTER 9
Challenges for the Public Health System

JESSIE WANG

The initial discovery of bovine spongiform encephalopathy (BSE) and its subsequent spread to humans through the consumption of contaminated meat led to a tremendous panic from the public, and ultimately called for many changes to be made to existing public health policies. It has been estimated that 750,000 BSE infected cattle were slaughtered and entered the United Kingdom food chain for human consumption between 1980 and 1999 (Ghani et al., 2000, as cited in Belay and Schonberger, 2005). Some European countries, such as Ireland, also suffered from BSE outbreaks in cattle as they had imported cattle and related meat products from the United Kingdom (Belay and Schonberger, 2005). In 1996, a new disease termed variant Creutzfeldt–Jakob disease (vCJD) was identified and the causative agent was later determined to be BSE infected cattle meat (Bruce et al., 1997). This prompted several public health measures to be put in place in order to reduce the risk of BSE transmission to humans, including the ban of certain cattle related materials in human food and the ban on the processing of cattle greater than 30 months old for human consumption (Smith and Bradley, 2003, as cited in Belay and Schonberger, 2005). The North American continent took appropriate measures to prevent the introduction of BSE, such as banning the importation of cattle or related cattle products from countries suffering from a BSE outbreak or at risk of a BSE outbreak (Kellar and Lees, 2003, as cited in Belay and Schonberger, 2005). In 2003 a case of an indegenous BSE infected cow was reported in Alberta, Canada, although meat from this cow did not enter the food chain for human consumption and no other related cattle herds were determined to be infected with BSE (Canadian Food Inspection Agency, 2003, as cited in Belay and Schonberger, 2005). Several months after, a BSE infected cow of Canadian origin was reported in the United States (Centers for Disease

Control and Prevention, 2003, as cited in Belay and Schonberger, 2005). Meat from this cow had entered the food chain, prompting a recall of meat and all other potentially infected products derived for the cattle (Centers for Disease Control and Prevention, 2003, as cited in Belay and Schonberger, 2005). Following this event, the USDA implemented several new measures to prevent the spread of BSE to humans, such as the removal of risk materials from cows greater than 30 months old, the banning of downer cows from being used in human food, and other measures to enhance the surveillance of BSE (Centers for Disease Control and Prevention, 2004, as cited in Belay and Schonberger, 2005).

Another prion disease, chronic wasting disease (CWD), is currently endemic in Saskatchewan, Canada and various parts of the United States (Williams et al., 2002). It is believed to have originated from north-central Colorado or from Wyoming in the United States (Williams and Young, 1980, as cited in Williams et al., 2002). CWD was first recognized during the 1960s in wildlife research facilities among mule deer, and later was found in elk from the same facilities (Williams and Young 1980, as cited in Williams et al., 2002). Due to the previous transmission of BSE to humans, there is concern that CWD could also spread to the human population. It is important to note that at the time, CWD does not appear to occur naturally outside of cervids. However, the possibility of CWD transmission has been demonstrated through lab studies. For instance, one study injected calves intracerebrally with a CWD prion agent isolated from mule deer (Hamir et al., 2001). Out of the 13 calves that were infected, 3 were successfully infected (Hamir et al., 2001). Due to these results, the possibility of CWD transmission cannot be ruled out. In regards to CWD transmission, there is specific concern that CWD could spread to various domestic animals that commonly interact with humans, which would effectively increase human exposure to the infectious prion agent (Belay et al., 2004). This is especially worrisome as the process of interspecies transmission could alter the properties of the prion agent, making them more infectious (Bartz et al., 1998). It has been previously demonstrated that although hamsters are resistant to infection by the scrapie prion agent carried by bovines, they are susceptible to scrapie after it is passaged through mice (Gibbs et al., 1996). This demonstrates that interspecies transmission may increase the infectivity of the prion agent by allowing it to gain the ability to infect a species that was previously resistant. A similar experiment has been done for the CWD prion agent in mule deer (Bartz et al., 1998). It has been observed that the CWD prion agent cannot be transmitted to hamsters directly from mules (Williams and Young, 1992, as cited in Bartz et al., 1998). However, hamsters are able to be infected with CWD when it is passaged through a ferret (Bartz et al., 1998). Additionally, the prion

66

agent becomes more pathogenic the further it is passaged through hamsters, indicating the selection of more infectious and dangerous prion strains (Bartz et al., 1998). These studies highlight the necessity of monitoring areas known to be endemic with CWD. Public health officials should pay close attention to these regions in order to ensure interspecies transmission does not occur, as this event may implicate increased risks of human transmission or pathogenicy.

Interspecies transmission may also be affected by how homologous the infecting prion agents are to the host prion proteins (Belay et al., 2004). This concept demonstrates that there exists a "species" barrier that must be overcome before successful transmission can occur (Belay et al., 2004). *In vitro* experiments have been done to assess how successfully the CWD prion agents can convert human prion proteins into the disease-causing isoform (Raymond et al., 2000). It was observed that such CWD prion agents can indeed convert human prions, but it does so at a very low rate (Raymond et al., 2000). Unfortunately, further studies to provide definitive evidence on whether transmission to humans is possible will be challenging, as experiments on transmission cannot be done on humans. The inability to perform these experiments leaves knowledge on how factors such as prion dose, route of infection, and prion stability within a host may affect infectivity (Raymond et al., 2000). However, considering that the BSE prion agent successfully transmitted to humans despite the species barrier between humans and cattle, the possibility of a similar transmission between humans and cervids could still be possible (Raymond et al., 2000). Thus, it is necessary to maintain precautionary measures in order to minimize the risk of such transmission. Both public health and wildlife agencies should keep up to date on where infected deer and elk are located and inform hunters accordingly (Belay et al., 2004). Hunters should also avoid handling or eating the brain and spinal cord of deer and elk from endemic regions as much as possible (Belay et al., 2004). Health Canada has also implemented measures that prevent CWD infected animals from entering the food chain or from being used in animal feed (Le Mauger, 2001, as cited in Kahn et al., 2004). Some Canadian provinces such as Manitoba, Saskatchewan, and Alberta require all slaughtered cervids to be held in the slaughterhouse until testing for CWD can be done (Kahn et al., 2004). These provinces, along with Ontario, Québec, and the Maritimes also issue velvet identification tags to help trace CWD if it is found after harvest is complete (Kahn et al., 2004).

Prions are often transmitted through the oral route, as seen in the Kuru disease that was spread through ritualistic cannibalism (Mathews, 1968). Indeed, the emergence of vCJD is thought to also have been transmitted orally through the consumption of food that has been contaminated by BSEs (Bruce et al., 1997). Thus, the risk of CJD spread may also pose difficulties in the oral health industry, where there is frequent use of medical instruments in oral cavities and thus a risk of prion spread when instruments are contaminated. At the time, there are no known cases of CJD that can be confidently linked to dental practices, although there have been two case reports with a possible connection to the dental sector (Will and Matthews, 1982; Arakawa et al., 1991, as cited in Smith et al., 2003). Despite this, TSEs still have implications on the dental industry due to the theoretical risks of iatrogenic transmission that have been demonstrated in laboratory studies. For instance, animal models have been used to measure the transmissibility of prions through dental instruments. In one study, gingival tissues of mice infected with scrapie were transferred to the gingival tissue of healthy mice using an unclean dental bur (Adams and Edgar, 1978). While mice traumatized with infected tissue did not exhibit symptoms or morphological features of scrapie disease, mice that were injected intraperitoneally did exhibit characteristics of scrapie disease (Adams and Edgar, 1978). Assuming that the prion agent responsible for CJD is similar to that of the scrapie agent used in this study in its mode of infectivity, it is possible that dental treatments could facilitate the transmission of prion diseases in humans as well (Adams and Edgar, 1978). Another model by Bourvis et al. estimates the risk of CJD transmission in endodontic practices, where instruments are often reused (2007). Under the assumption that dental pulp is able to be infected by prions, their model identifies a non-zero risk of prion transmission from one patient to another (Bourvis et al., 2007).

A major complication that prions pose in the public health sector is related to their resistance towards many forms of decontamination, such as ionizing, ultraviolet, or microwave radiation (Taylor, 1999). Prions are also resistant to heat, and thus cannot be easily inactivated by autoclaving (Taylor, 1999). Certain methods of heat sterilization may actually fix contaminants on the instruments, intensifying the problem (Letters et al., 2005). It has also been observed that the effectiveness of autoclaving declines with increasing temperature for some prion populations (Taylor, 1999). This is likely due to the fact that some subpopulations of prions are very resistant to heat, making them difficult to kill just by increasing the duration or temperature of autoclaving (Taylor, 1999). As such, many methods of chemical or heat based methods of decontamination will likely also damage medical instruments. This is especially problematic in dental practices, as prions are resistant to a large majority of the commonly used disinfectants in these practices (Smith et al., 2003). In addition, dental instruments are small and have intricate designs, making them challenging to clean (Smith et al., 2002). This

68

issue is exacerbated by the fact that many dental practitioners may reuse instruments that are labeled as single use by the manufacturer (Letters et al., 2005). A questionnaire sent to 25 dental practices found that no practitioners switch endodontic files after each patient, and 84% of practitioners do treat endodontic files as single-use due to the cost implications (Letters et al., 2005). Due to the reuse of these instruments, tissue debris containing infectious contaminants may build up over time, especially when methods such as heat sterilization are used (Letters et al., 2005). These studies suggest that endodontic instruments cannot be reliably disinfected and reused, underscoring the importance of implementing proper policies and recommendations for dental practitioners in order to prevent the transmission of prion diseases (Letters et al., 2005). Additionally, these studies also highlight issues regarding regulatory policies in place for reviewing the efficacy of decontamination procedures provided by dental instrument manufacturers and the funding of endodontic procedures in dental practices (Letters et al., 2005). The development of new more reliable methods of sterilization will remain a challenge for the public health industry, especially given the resistant nature of prions.

Several measures have been put in place to ensure that prions do not spread through dental instruments. Healthcare practitioners are given precautions to use single-use disposable items as often as possible, to discard items that are difficult to clean after a single use, and to keep medical instruments as moist as possible in order to stop the drying of tissues onto the devices (Kohn et al., 2003). For instruments that are not single-use, it is recommended to autoclave the instruments at 134°C for 18 minutes (Kohn et al., 2003). Although this method of sterilization does not eliminate all residual infectivity, it should greatly decrease the risk of secondary infections (Bourvis et al., 2007). More specific measures should be put in place when performing invasive procedures, especially when they concern patients deemed to be at risk (Shushma et al., 2016). These patients are recommended to attend specialist clinics or hospitals, and all dental instruments used in their procedures are to be incinerated. Before incineration or disposal, these instruments should be contained using cover sheets in order to minimize contamination with the environment or the work area (Shushma et al., 2016). During dental treatments with these patients, the activation of water lines should be minimized as much as possible in order to prevent the retraction of prions in oral fluids (Shushma et al., 2016). Lastly, patients at risk or patients that have been infected with a prion disease are recommended to be scheduled at the end of the day to allow more thorough decontamination of the work area (Shushma et al., 2016).

Another method of iatrogenic vCJD transmission is through blood transfusions. The concern surrounding this route of iatrogenic transmission was explored in 1999, when the FDA implemented a policy that would exclude blood donors who have spent time in the United Kingdom or other European countries that were affected by the vCJD outbreak (Gottlieb, 1999). During this time, there was no evidence that bloodborne transmission of vCJD was possible outside of laboratory experiments, but the theoretical risks of vCJD spread was enough to warrant the implementation of preventative measures (Gottlieb, 1999). In 2002, vCJD was reported in a man residing in the United Kingdom who had received a blood transfusion from another patient that died of vCJD 2 years earlier (Llewelyn et al., 2004). This case emphasizes the importance of epidemiological surveillance systems when trying to assess the risk of iatrogenic transmission of vCJD (Llewelyn et al., 2004). Also of note is that before 1998, plasma from donors who later developed vCJD were used for the production of fractionated plasma products, and such products have been exposed to many individuals who have not been infected (Llewelyn et al., 2004). Studies have shown that several steps throughout the plasma fractionation process may remove prion agents and thus reduce the infectivity of these products (Foster et al., 2000, as cited in Llewelyn et al., 2004). However, the Transmissible Spongiform Encephalopathies Advisory Committee agreed that the labelling of products derived from the plasma of donors, such as albumin, should be recommended in order to reflect the possibility of vCJD transmission (U. S. Food and Drug Administration, 2010).

In the future, sporadic cases of BSE may continue to pose a challenge to the public health sector, irrespective of how much the risk of iatrogenic transmission is minimized. For instance, a novel sporadic prion disease termed variably proteinase-sensitive prionopathy (PSPr) has been identified (Gambetti et al., 2008). Additionally, interspecies transmission could also pose a challenge by creating novel animal carriers that are able to infect humans. Thus, both preventative measures regarding iagogeric transmission and continued surveillance of both human prion disorders and prion disorders epidemic regions are necessary to prevent escalation of prion spread. Future studies on how prion infectivity differs depending on the route of infection and dose of prion agent needed for successful infection will be helpful in determining the risks that prions pose on the public health sector.

CHAPTER 10

Skepticism surrounding Prions and its Diseases

JAMIE JOHNSON

Since the late 19th century, infectious diseases were proven to be caused by either bacteria, fungi, parasites, or viruses, so when the discovery of prions as a disease-causing agent was brought to light, naturally there was some skepticism. How can something that is not technically "alive" cause a disease or an infection?

Nobel Prize winner, Stanley Prusiner, admitted that new ideas in science are not always correct, so doubt in their validity is to be expected. When he discovered and coined the term "prion" critics went as far as accusing him of wanting fame more than scientific answers. He endeavored to focus on finding those answers rather than entertain notions of naysayers and from that point on, he refused to talk to reporters (Corbyn, 2014).

In 1967, scrapie was first hypothesized to be caused by a protein agent, by scientists Alper, Griffith, and Pattison. This was considered a radical idea at the time because it went against the central dogma of molecular biology, first described by Crick in 1958, which dictates that nucleic acid (DNA or RNA) is needed for replication of an organism. In other words, a protein contains no such genetic material necessary to copy itself so how could it thus cause disease or infection like other DNA/RNA-containing agents that can replicate to infect? Prusiner further argued that scrapie was caused *only* by protein and the protein-only hypothesis was born (Zabel & Reid, 2015). Since this idea was new and went against the standards of how microorganisms can infect and cause disease, skepticism was inevitable.

Gary Taubes, the writer of the Discover magazine article that accused Prusiner of being on a quest for fame, also criticized him for attempting to stop publications that went against his theories. Taubes points out that one of the experiments led by Prusiner and Weissmann provided support that the prion was not in fact the infectious agent because of the presence of mRNA in the protein. This contradicts claims by Prusiner that there is no nucleic acid in the prions (Liu, 2011). Taubes (1986), goes on to say that all Prusiner did was give a name to something that was already known and that he named this without proof of its existence.

Ledford (2007) reminds us that despite years of research supporting the protein-only or prion hypothesis, and a Nobel Prize for the discovery notwithstanding, arguments are still being made against it. She suggests the mere mention of the name Laura Manuelidis is enough to upset supporters of the widely accepted and proven hypothesis. She summarizes an article published in the Proceedings of the National Academy of Sciences written by Dr. Laura Manuelidis, a neuropathologist from Yale University, stating that demonstrating how difficult it is to narrow down the cause of a disease does not negate the generally acknowledged protein-only hypothesis. From Dr. Laura Manuelidis' perspective, there is a viral component to the transmission of prion diseases despite research results confirming that is not the case (Ledford, 2007).

According to Charles Weissmann, a molecular biologist from the Scripps Research facility in Florida, Manuelidis has yet to prove her results of a viral component are the cause of prion infection and has also not proven that these particles do not contain the prion protein (Ledford, 2007). However, Hendricks (2019) states that Manuelidis claims there has been proof of no detectable prions in virus particles. She further asserts that there is no proof that a protein can, in fact, be infectious because they do not contain nucleic acid and cannot replicate themselves a million times over as a result, like other infectious agents can (Hendricks, 2019). In an article for Science titled The Prion Heretic, Manuelidis admits that although she is adamant that a virus causes these diseases, she has no proof of this claim other than her belief that the rules of infectious diseases cannot be bent to accommodate new theories and just because no one has found these hypothetical viruses does not mean they do not exist (Couzin-Frankel, 2011). Soto (2011) says, "the idea that prions consist of viruses or any other type of conventional micro-organism is simply untenable" (para. 7).

It was discovered that cellular prion protein (PrPC), a normal cellular protein, is needed to cause a prion disease. Several experiments were done by different scientists that supported this hypothesis, but the skeptics did not stop at criticizing the very idea that a protein can cause disease. They claimed that the PrPC used in those experiments to generate new prion infections came from animals who were already infected with transmissible spongiform encephalopathies (TSE) virus (Zabel & Reid, 2015).

The argument against the prion hypothesis is easy to make because there are some of Prusiner's experiments that have not been replicated by other labs. Robert Rohwer, a neurovirologist from Baltimore, Maryland points out the mice experiments in Prusiner's work failed to produce the prion in a normal mouse; the mice used were already predisposed to developing the prion disease (Ledford, 2007). Manuelidis used this argument as support that prions are not infectious, stating that there are no replicated results in support of the prion hypothesis among experiments numbering in the thousands (Hendricks, 2019). However, in 2010, an experiment was performed by Jiyan Ma, a biochemist from Ohio State University, in normal mice that produced a disease-causing prion (Couzin-Frankel, 2011).

Manuelidis states that disease is caused by infectious agents and not transmitted, but later a seemingly contradictory statement is made regarding the disappearance of kuru. She says that kuru disappeared in conjunction with the end of cannibalism practices, but this begs the question of how the tribe members contracted kuru if not by transmission? She states that the prion hypothesis is refuted because its basic principle stipulates a spontaneous appearance of the disease (Hendricks, 2019). In an interview with Science, Couzin-Frankel (2011) noted that attempts to have Manuelidis explain why she was skeptical was challenging because her reasons were not easy to understand. Manuelidis was quoted as saying, "I can't think in a straight sentence" (Couzin-Frankel, 2011, p. 4).

Arguing against a widely accepted and scientifically proven hypothesis does not come without consequences. Manuelidis has been screamed at in meetings and walked out on in lectures (Couzin-Frankel, 2011). She complains being published in top journals has proven difficult due to her disbelief in prions (Ledford, 2007) and finds reviews of her work that are based on personal attacks (Couzin-Frankel, 2011).

Manuelidis is not the only scientist refuting the prion hypothesis. Dr. Frank Bastian, a neuropathologist from the University of New Orleans, claims that the cause of both scrapie and chronic wasting disease is not prions and asserts to have linked both diseases to spiroplasma bacteria-carrying hay mites. Bastian claims that this bacterium (various strains, depending on the disease) is present in all transmissible spongiform encephalopathies (TSE) diseases and what is not present in all of them is prions. He says he has not been able to duplicate or further research his results because the funding for TSE research is awarded to those studying prions and not bacteria (Sorenson, 2019). He further asserts that a common antibiotic, tetracycline, can cure scrapie (Hendricks, 2019).

In perhaps, the most controversial statement made, Bastian recently told Steve Sorenson of Deer and Deer Hunting (2019), "up to 15 percent of all Alzheimer's disease deaths might be misclassified cases of Creutzfeldt-Jakob disease" (para.1). If Bastian's theories are correct, and if there was funding available for further research, then chronic wasting disease (CWD) could be prevented with vaccines and this research could be used to find treatments for other neurodegenerative diseases in both humans and animals (Sorenson, 2019). However, other scientists claim to have proven Bastian's results and research wrong. Wildlife biologist, Merril Cook says, "It's been over 15 years since he first made those claims, yet no other researcher has been able to reproduce his findings," (Cope et al. 2019). Scientist Brent Race, failed to reproduce Bastian's results. In fact, his results confirmed the prion hypothesis. Bastian maintains that the results did not stem from a replication of his work, but rather they were biased by those who support the prion hypothesis (Cope et al. 2019).

Krysten Schuler, a wildlife disease ecologist, examines 6 points of evidence that contradict Bastian's bacteria theory and offers explanations for each that show support in favour of the prion hypothesis. First, she suggests that if chronic wasting disease (CWD) were bacterial in nature, there should be an immune response when it enters the body. Much like when you catch the common cold virus, your body immediately begins to fight it off and signs of infection are present such as fever. No such signs are evident in CWD. Second, bacteria and viruses can be killed, prions cannot. If CWD were bacterial, it would stand to reason that it could be cured. Third, Bastian's studies of prions binding to soil has actually provided proof that CWD is caused by prions. The process to purify an environment from prions is to remove contaminated equipment or decontaminate it, ensure the paddock is not used for at least two years, and restock it with animals who are free of CWD. However, since prions can bind to soil particles and remain there for years, the evidence showed that even a "clean" environment can produce the disease in animals who were not otherwise exposed. Fourth, since normal cell (non-infectious) prions are needed to create infectious prions, experiments have been done in animals that eliminated these normal cells to see if they were able to get a transmissible spongiform encephalopathy (TSE) any other way. The results showed they could not, which supports the protein-hypothesis. Fifth, studies have shown that TSE diseases can be caused using synthetic

74

prions. Lastly, and perhaps most convincingly, no test has been able to confirm the presence of bacteria in an infected animal. Since viruses and bacteria contain the necessary nucleic acid (DNA or RNA) to cause disease, proof of this DNA or RNA should be evident in tissue examination. No genetic sequencing has been found to support the presence of the spiroplasma bacteria Bastian claims to be the cause (Schuler, 2019).

It is not just scientists who have something to say about prions. John Mark Purdy, an organic farmer from England had his own theories about the cause of BSE bovine spongiform encephalopathy (BSE). He did not argue against the protein agent being the cause of the disease, but rather he thinks the reason the proteins misfold is because of a chemical used to treat cows infested with warble fly. He says they are not infected through transmission by ingestion of infected meat and bone meal used to feed the cows (BBC, 1998). He also theorized that exposure to metals such as manganese and copper played a role in the misfolding of proteins. According to Purdy's obituary, his theories were ultimately proven incorrect and unsubstantiated through experiments by the Medical Research Council in 1995. Further research was completed and the conclusion that BSE was caused by ingestion of contaminated feed was ultimately reached. Purdy passed on before he could continue his own research. He wanted to find the answers that explain why countries who used the same bone meal imported from the UK did not have instances of BSE in their livestock (The Independent, 2007).

The controversy and skepticism do not end with the protein-only hypothesis. Since the very definition of a prion stipulates that it causes infectious disease and that these diseases are transmissible, referring to certain neurodegenerative diseases such as Alzheimer's in these terms is not something all scientists will agree to (Zabel & Reid, 2015). Dr. David R. Brown, a neuroscientist, has done extensive research on prions. His research on metals in relation to prion disease was pushed into the spotlight as a result of the passion Mark Purdy showed for his own theories on the cause of BSE in relation to metal poisoning. Brown (2010) summarizes numerous studies confirming that the prion protein binds with copper and further asserts that copper can both cause and prevent proteins from misforming. Aside from copper, other metals such as zinc, iron, and manganese can also bind to the protein and that the exposure to, or infectivity of these metals in the brain could be associated with the development of a prion disease (Brown, 2010). Brown (2010), states, "while there has been some recent speculation that other neurodegenerative disorders could be transmissible, this has no basis in observed fact" (para.1). The presence of manganese in proteins was documented in the frontal cortex, cerebellum, and in the blood those with Creutzfeldt–Jakob Disease (CJD), a known prion disease. This is not the case with patients of Alzheimer's or Parkinson's disease (Brown, 2010). What this seems to indicate is that because CJD is a prion disease found in humans and manganese is not found in other neurodegenerative diseases in humans, those diseases (Alzheimer's or Parkinson's) are not necessarily caused by prions. These recent results also suggest that it is not necessarily environmental exposure to manganese that causes the prion disease, but it is possible that the disease is responsible for the manganese staying attached to the proteins (Brown, 2010).

So why has there been so much controversy and skepticism? In a doctoral dissertation, Patricia Liu notes that skeptics of the prion hypothesis had the results of their studies published only in scientific or speciality journals. These publications are not accessible to everyone so important studies that oppose and potentially have evidence against the prion hypothesis do not see the light of day in the mainstream. News articles and other popular literature seem to favour writings that support Prusiner's theories. She also points out that perhaps Prusiner's theories would be taken more seriously by specialists in the scientific community if they were also published in these same journals as opposed to magazines and other popular news media outlets. Charles Weissmann, who conducted experiments with Pruisner, was not 100% convinced that the prion found to cause scrapie was not viral in nature, yet his reservations were never published in the media with Prusiner's work supporting his hypothesis (Liu, 2011). She further explains the reason Prusiner's results are subject to various interpretations is because they were largely experimental and that, "scientists and the public's openness to certain interpretations are what determine the success of a scientific theory (p. 42). She further cites an article that explains that ideas that are not widely accepted by skeptics are accepted by people who do not have extensive knowledge in that particular field and that these individuals believe these ideas to be the truth. In other words, the average person is more likely to believe what the media tells them is fact. It would be reasonable to assume that in turn, the ideas are promoted, funded, and written about more in popular media, and thus the cycle continues. It was the article written for Discover in 1986, by Gary Taubes that silenced Prusiner for some time, but he has many other supporters of his hypothesis who speak out against the skepticism.

With ongoing research, sometimes more questions are generated than answered. Soto (2011) listed several questions regarding prions that remain unanswered. A normal protein PrPc is misfolded into PrPSc (the infectious protein), but are there any other factors that make this protein infectious? This question remains to be answered. He also asks how PrPSc induces brain degeneration. Brown (2010) points out that in order to understand how disease is caused by PrPSc the molecular biology of the non-pathogenic proteins must be studied. With a lengthy incubation period in humans, these diseases are not often seen in patients under 60 which gives rise to another unanswered question: can these cellular mutations or misfolding of an otherwise normal cell which exist in everyone, be caused by cellular aging (Brown, 2010)? Iyer (2004) asks how prions reach the brain once transmitted into the body, how are normal cells transformed into the misfolded infectious proteins and how do these infectious proteins cause neurodegeneration? The function of PrP has also yet to have been determined and scientists suggest that once it has, we will have a better understanding of prion diseases (Legname, 2017).

Soto (2011) notes another unanswered question: what is the 3-dimensional structure of PrPSc? Wille & Requena (2018) seem to have answered this by defining its structure as a four-rung β-solenoid, but they admit that without a high-resolution examination of PrPSc there are still unanswered questions regarding its structure.

As we have learned, there was a lot of skepticism surrounding the prion theory because its structure does not contain the necessary genetic material to replicate and to infect. Stanley Prusiner, prion discoverer and creator of the protein-only or prion hypothesis has received much attention in the media regarding his discoveries and research, not all of it in support of his theory and some of it negative. It seems as though the skepticism lies mainly in the idea that something that has no components of either a virus or bacteria can cause neurodegenerative disease in animals and humans alike. The skepticism has been somewhat limited to scientific journals, while the opposite is true for those who support the theory; views in favour of it are highly publicized in popular media and research on the idea that prion diseases are caused only by prions are funded more easily than research that supports an alternate theory. For almost every point either for or against the theory, there is a counterpoint, but it seems as though it was the skeptics who were actually silenced. As with any new scientific discovery, there has and will likely always be many questions we cannot readily answer.

CONCLUSION
Future Directions: Where is Prion Science Headed?

JANVI BEDI

The result of Stanley Prusiner's breakthrough discovery altered the course of molecular biology, and opened up pathways to a multitude of directions (Aguzzi & Cecco, 2020). Although there have been remarkable strides made in the discovery and understanding of prions, much remains elusive.

The list of unanswered questions includes mystery around its physical nature, the biochemical basis of prion strains, the factors that promote prion infections, amongst many others (Aguzzi & Heikenwalder, 2006).

Perhaps the main direction of prions science points towards the role of the protein-only prion replication hypothesis which describes how a pathogenic conformation of a prion protein is capable of inducing a native folded protein into a misfolded, pathogenic protein in a process that involves modification of the secondary and tertiary structures of the protein (Guest et al., 2011). Currently, there is accumulating evidence that there may be a similar protein misfolding mechanism for proteins involved in diseases such as Alzheimers and Parkinsons (Guest et al., 2011). In turn, the implication of such evidence suggests that the template-directed misfolding mechanisms of prions could be at the epicenter of understanding many diseases which affect the central nervous system (Guest et al., 2011). This example is one of many which implicates the importance of understanding the functions of prions in terms of a variety of diseases and points the scientific field towards this type of investigation. The understanding of prions has amassed great knowledge in the scientific field. Through the development of new technologies and research into its mechanism and pathogenesis, the future of uncovering its mysteries remains bright.

REFERENCES

Acevedo-Morantes, C. Y., & Wille, H. (2014). The structure of human prions: from biology to structural models-considerations and pitfalls. *Viruses, 6*(10), 3875–3892. https://doi.org/10.3390/v6103875

Adams, D. H., & Edgar, W. M. (1978). Transmission of agent of Creutzfeldt-Jakob disease. *British Medical Journal, 1*(6118), 987. https://www.ncbi.nlm.nih.gov/pmc/articles/PMC1603797/?page=1

Aguzzi, A., & Calella, A. M. (2009). Prions: Protein Aggregation and Infectious Diseases. *Physiological Reviews, 89*(4), 1105–1152. https://doi.org/10.1152/physrev.00006.2009

Aguzzi, A., & Cecco, E. D. (2020). Shifts and drifts in prion science. *Science, 370*(6512), 32–34. https://doi.org/10.1126/science.abb8577

Aguzzi, A., & Heikenwalder, M. (2006). Pathogenesis of prion diseases: Current status and future outlook. *Nature Reviews Microbiology, 4*(10), 765–775. https://doi.org/10.1038/nrmicro1492

Alberta Prion Research Institute. (n.d.). *Why Prion Research?*. http://prioninstitute.ca/content/why-prion-research

Alper, T., Cramp, W. A., Haig, D. A., & Clarke, M. C. (1967). Does the agent of scrapie replicate without nucleic acid? *Nature, 214*, 764-766. https://doi.org/10.1038/214764a0

Alpers, M. P. (2008). Review. The epidemiology of kuru: Monitoring the epidemic from its peak to its end. *Philosophical Transactions of the Royal Society of London. Series B, Biological Sciences, 363*(1510), 3707–3713. https://doi.org/10.1098/rstb.2008.0071

Alzheon, Inc. (n.d.). Alzheon Appoints Nobel Laureate Stanley B. Prusiner, MD, Retrieved from: https://alzheon.com/alzheon-appoints-nobel-laureate-stan-ley-b-prusiner-md-chair-scientific-advisory-board/#:~:text=Prusiner%20currently%20serves%20as%20the,scientists%2C%20clinicians%20and%20drug%20developers

Atalay, F. Ö., Tolunay, Ş., Özgün, G., Bekar, A., & Zarifoğlu, M. (2015). Creutzfeldt-Jakob disease: Report of four cases and review of the literature. *Turk Patoloji Dergisi, 31*(2), 148–152. https://doi.org/10.5146/tjpath.2013.01195

Bartz, J. C., Marsh, R. F., McKenzie, D. I., & Aiken, J. M. (1998). The Host Range of Chronic Wasting Disease Is Altered on Passage in Ferrets. *Virology, 251*(2), 297–301. https://doi.org/10.1006/viro.1998.9427

Basler, K., Oesch, B., Scott, M., Westaway, D., Wälchli, M., Groth, D.F, McKinley, M.P., Prusiner, S.B, Weissmann, C. (1986). Scrapie and cellular PrP isoforms are encoded by the same chromosomal gene. *Cell, 46*(3), 417-428. doi:10.1016/0092-8674(86)90662-8

BBC. (1998, April 2). *UK | Farmer says chemicals cause BSE*. BBC News. http://news.bbc.co.uk/2/hi/uk_news/72866.stm.

Belay, E. D., & Schonberger, L. B. (2005). The public health impact of prion diseases. *Annu. Rev. Public Health, 26*, 191-212. https://doi.org/10.1146/annurev.publhealth.26.021304.144536

Belay, E. D., Maddox, R. A., Williams, E. S., Miller, M. W., Gambetti, P., & Schonberger, L. B. (2004). Chronic Wasting Disease and Potential Transmission to Humans. *Emerging Infectious Diseases, 10*(6), 977–984. https://doi.org/10.3201/eid1006.031082

Bennett, J. H., Rhodes, F. A., & Robson, H. N. (1959). A Possible Genetic Basis for Kuru. *American Journal of Human Genetics, 11*(2 Pt 1), 169–187.

Bessen, R. A., & Marsh, R. F. (1994). Distinct PrP properties suggest the molecular basis of strain variation in transmissible mink encephalopathy. *Journal of Virology, 68*(12), 7859-7868. doi:10.1128/jvi.68.12.7859-7868.1994

Bolton, D. (2004). Prions, the Protein Hypothesis, and Scientific Revolutions. https://www.researchgate.net/publication/235220355_Prions_the_Protein_Hypothesis_and_Scientific_Revolutions

Borchelt, D. R., Scott, M., Taraboulos, A., Stahl, N., & Prusiner, S. B. (1990). Scrapie And Cellular Prion Proteins Differ In Their Kinetics Of Synthesis And Topology In Cultured Cells. *Journal of Neuropathology and Experimental Neurology, 49*(3), 311. doi:10.1097/00005072-199005000-00156

Bourvis, N., Boelle, P.-Y., Cesbron, J.-Y., & Valleron, A.-J. (2007). Risk Assessment of Transmission of Sporadic Creutzfeldt-Jakob Disease in Endodontic Practice in Absence of Adequate Prion Inactivation. *PLoS ONE, 2*(12), e1330. https://doi.org/10.1371/journal.pone.0001330

Brandner, S. (2003). CNS pathogenesis of prion diseases. *British Medical Bulletin, 66*(1), 131–139. https://doi.org/10.1093/bmb/66.1.131

Brandner, S., Whitfield, J., Boone, K., Puwa, A., O'Malley, C., Linehan, J. M., Joiner, S., Scaravilli, F., Calder, I., Alpers, M. P., Wadsworth, J. D. F., & Collinge, J. (2008). Central and peripheral pathology of kuru: Pathological analysis of a recent case and comparison with other forms of human prion disease. *Philosophical Transactions of the Royal Society B: Biological Sciences, 363*(1510), 3755–3763. https://doi.org/10.1098/rstb.2008.0091

BrightFocus Foundation. (2016). *Dr. Stanley Prusiner Acceptance Speech.* [Video file]. Retrieved from: https://www.youtube.com/watch?v=dxLqSUn1IOg

BrightFocus Foundation. (n.d.). Stanley B. Prusiner, MD, Honorary Member. In *Board.* Retrieved from: https://www.brightfocus.org/bio/stanley-b-prusiner-md

BrightFocus Foundation. (n.d.). Stanley Prusiner, MD. *In Notable Researchers.* Retrieved from: https://www.brightfocus.org/research/notable-researchers#prusiner

Brown, D. 2010. Prions and manganese: A maddening beast, *Metallomics*, Volume 3, Issue 3, March 2011, Pages 229–238, https://doi.org/10.1039/c0mt00047g

Brown, P., Will, R. G., Bradley, R., Asher, D. M. & Detwiler, L. (2001). Bovine spongiform encephalopathy and variant Creutzfeldt-Jakob Disease: Background, evolution, and current concerns. *Emerging Infectious Diseases, 7*(1), 6-16. https://doi.org/10.3201/eid0701.700006.

Bruce, M. E., Will, R. G., Ironside, J. W., McConnell, I., Drummond, D., Suttie, A., McCardle, L., Chree, A., Hope, J., Birkett, C., Cousens, S., Fraser, H., & Bostock, C. J. (1997). Transmissions to mice indicate that "new variant" CJD is caused by the BSE agent. *Nature, 389*(6650), 498–501. https://doi.org/10.1038/39057

Bruner, R. (2020, August 15). *Prions.* https://bio.libretexts.org/@go/page/407

Büeler, H., Aguzzi, A., Sailer, A., Greiner, R., Autenried, P., Aguet, M., & Weissmann, C. (1993). Mice devoid of PrP are resistant to scrapie. *Cell, 73*(7), 1339-1347. doi:10.1016/0092-8674(93)90360-3

Büeler, H., Fischer, M., Lang, Y., Bluethmann, H., Lipp, H., Dearmond, S. J., Pruisner, S. B., Aguet, M., Weissmann, C. (1992). Normal development and behaviour of mice lacking the neuronal cell-surface PrP protein. *Nature, 356*(6370), 577-582. doi:10.1038/356577a0

Carlson, G. A., Westaway, D., Dearmond, S. J., Peterson-Torchia, M., & Prusiner, S. B. (1989). Primary structure of prion protein may modify scrapie isolate properties. *Proceedings of the National Academy of Sciences, 86*(19), 7475-7479. doi:10.1073/pnas.86.19.7475

Caughey, B., & Raymond, G. (1991). The scrapie-associated form of PrP is made from a cell surface precursor that is both protease- and phospholipase-sensitive. *Journal of Biological Chemistry, 266*(27), 18217-18223. doi:10.1016/s0021-9258(18)55257-1

Caughey, B., Kocisko, D. A., Raymond, G. J., & Lansbury, P. T. (1995). Aggregates of scrapie-associated prion protein induce the cell-free conversion of protease-sensitive prion protein to the protease-resistant state. *Chemistry & Biology, 2*(12), 807-817. doi:10.1016/1074-5521(95)90087-x

Center for Food Safety. (n.d.). Timeline of Mad Cow Disease Outbreaks. Retrieved from: https://www.centerforfoodsafety.org/issues/1040/mad-cow-disease/timeline-mad-cow-disease-outbreaks

Centers for Disease Control and Prevention (2018, October 9). Prion diseases. https://www.cdc.gov/prions/index.html

Chandra, S., Mahadevan, A., & Shankar, S. K. (2019). Familial CJD- A Brief Commentary. *Annals of Indian Academy of Neurology, 22*(4), 462–463. https://doi.org/10.4103/aian.AIAN_508_19

Chesebro, B. (2003). Introduction to the transmissible spongiform encephalopathies or prion diseases. *British Medical Bulletin, 66*, 1–20. https://doi.org/10.1093/bmb/66.1.1

Clift, K., Guthrie, K., Klee, E. W., Boczek, N., Cousin, M., Blackburn, P., & Atwal, P. (2016). Familial Creutzfeldt-Jakob Disease: Case report and role of genetic counseling in post mortem testing. Prion, 10(6), 502–506. https://doi.org/1 0.1080/19336896.2016.1254858

Cobb, N. J., & Surewicz, W. K. (2009). Prion Diseases and Their Biochemical Mechanisms. *Biochemistry, 48*(12), 2574–2585. https://doi.org/10.1021/bi900108v

Colby, D. W., & Prusiner, S. B. (2011). Prions. *Cold Spring Harbor Perspectives in Biology, 3*(1). doi:10.1101/cshperspect.a006833

Collee, J. G., Bradley, R., & Liberski, P. P. (2006). Variant CJD (vCJD) and bovine spongiform encephalopathy (BSE): 10 and 20 years on: part 2. *Folia Neuropathologica, 44*(2), 102–110.

Collinge, J., & Clarke, A. R. (2007). A general model of prion strains and their pathogenicity. *Science, 318*(5852), 930-936. https://doi.org/10.1126/science.1138718

Collinge, J., Sidle, K. C., Meads, J., Ironside, J., & Hill, A. F. (1996). Molecular analysis of prion strain variation and the aetiology of new variant CJD. *Nature, 383*(6602), 685-690. doi:10.1038/383685a0

Collinge, J., Whittington, M. A., Sidle, K. C., Smith, C. J., Palmer, M. S., Clarke, A. R., & Jefferys, J. G. (1994). *Nature, 370*(6487), 295-297. doi:10.1038/370295a0

Collins, S., McLean, C. A., & Masters, C. L. (2001). Gerstmann-Sträussler-Scheinker syndrome,fatal familial insomnia, and kuru. *Journal of Clinical Neuroscience: Official Journal of the Neurosurgical Society of Australasia, 8*(5), 387–397. https://doi.org/10.1054/jocn.2001.0919 Colorado State University. (n.d.). *Prion Basics*

Cope, B., Garbo, B., Cleveland, B., & Kibler, D. (2019, September 5). *Has LSU researcher found a cure for CWD? Scientists say, 'no'.* Mississippi Sportsman. https://www.ms-sportsman.com/hunting/deer-hunting/has-lsu-researcher-found-a-cure-for-cwd-scientists-say-no/.

Corbyn , Z. (2014, May 24). *Stanley Prusiner: 'A Nobel prize doesn't wipe the scepticism away'.* The Guardian. https://www.theguardian.com/science/2014/may/25/stanley-prusiner-neurologist-nobel-doesnt-wipe-scepticism-away

Couzin-Frankel, J. (2011). The Prion Heretic. Science, 332(6033), 1024-1027. http://www.jstor.org/stable/27977920

Das, A. S., & Zou, W.-Q. (2016). Prions: Beyond a Single Protein. *Clinical Microbiology Reviews, 29*(3), 633–658. https://doi.org/10.1128/CMR.00046-15

Derkatch, I.L., Bradley, M.E., Hong J.Y., Liebman, S.W. (2001). Prions affect the appearance of other prions: the story of [PIN(+)]. *Cell 106*(2):171-82. https://doi.org/10.1016/s0092-8674(01)00427-5

Diagnostic Criteria. (2019, January 24). Retrieved from https://www.cdc.gov/prions/cjd/diagnostic-criteria.html

Dickinson, A. G., Meikle, V. M., & Fraser, H. (1968). Identification of a gene which controls the incubation period of some strains of scrapie agent in mice. *Journal of Comparative Pathology, 78*(3), 293-299. https://doi.org/10.1016/0021-9975(68)90005-4

Dietz, K., Raddatz, G., Wallis, J., Müller, N., Zerr, I., Duerr, H.-P., Lefèvre, H., Seifried, E., & Löwer, J. (2007). Blood Transfusion and Spread of Variant Creutzfeldt-Jakob Disease. *Emerging Infectious Diseases, 13*(1), 89–96. https://doi.org/10.3201/eid1301.060396

Donnelly, C. A., Ferguson, N. M., Ghani, A. C., & Anderson, R. M. (2002). Implications of BSE infection screening data for the scale of the British BSE epidemic and current European infection levels. *Proceedings of the Royal Society of London. Series B: Biological Sciences, 269*(1506), 2179–2190. https://doi.org/10.1098/rspb.2002.2156

Duke University. (n.d.). *How prions came to be: A brief history.* Infectious Disease: Superbugs, Science, & Society. Retrieved May 3, 2021, from https://sites.duke.edu/superbugs/module-6/prions-mad-cow-disease-when-proteins-go-bad/how-prions-came-to-be-a-brief-history/

Fatal Familial Insomnia. (2020, November 18). Retrieved from https://rarediseases.org/rare-diseases/fatal-familial-insomnia/#:~:text=Fatal familial insomnia (FFI) is,significant physical and mental deterioration.

Gabriel, J. M., Oesch, B., Kretzschmar, H., Scott, M., & Prusiner, S. B. (1992). Molecular cloning of a candidate chicken prion protein. *Proceedings of the National Academy of Sciences, 89*(19), 9097-9101. doi:10.1073/pnas.89.19.9097

Gambetti, P., Dong, Z., Yuan, J., Xiao, X., Zheng, M., Alshekhlee, A., Castellani, R., Cohen, M., Barria, M. A., Gonzalez-Romero, D., Belay, E. D., Schonberger, L. B., Marder, K., Harris, C., Burke, J. R., Montine, T., Wisniewski, T., Dickson, D. W., Soto, C., & Hulette, C. M. (2008). A Novel Human Disease with Abnormal Prion Protein Sensitive to Protease. *Annals of Neurology, 63*(6), 697–708. https://doi.org/10.1002/ana.21420

Gasset, M., Baldwin, M. A., Lloyd, D. H., Gabriel, J. M., Holtzman, D. M., Cohen, F., Fletterick, R., Prusiner, S. B. (1992). Predicted alpha-helical regions of the prion protein when synthesized as peptides form amyloid. *Proceedings of the National Academy of Sciences, 89*(22), 10940-10944. doi:10.1073/pnas.89.22.10940

Gerstmann-Sträussler-Scheinker Disease. (2019, February 23). Retrieved from https://rarediseases.org/rare-diseases/gerstmann-straussler-scheinker-disease/

Gibb, B. J. (2007). *The Rough Guide to The Brain*. New York, USA: Penguin Books Ltd.

Gibbs C.J., Safar J., Sulima M.P., Bacote A.E., San Martin R.A. (1996) Transmission of Sheep and Goat Strains of Scrapie from Experimentally Infected Cattle to Hamsters and Mice. In: Gibbs C.J. (eds) *Bovine Spongiform Encephalopathy* (pp. 84-91). Springer, New York, NY. https://doi.org/10.1007/978-1-4612-2406-8_6

Gorodinsky, A., & Harris, D. A. (1995). Glycolipid-anchored proteins in neuroblastoma cells form detergent-resistant complexes without caveolin. *Journal of Cell Biology, 129*(3), 619-627. doi:10.1083/jcb.129.3.619

Gottlieb, S. (1999). FDA bans blood donation by people who have lived in UK. *BMJ : British Medical Journal, 319*(7209), 535. https://www.ncbi.nlm.nih.gov/pmc/articles/PMC1116429/

Griffith, J. S. (1967). Self-replication and scrapie. Nature, 215, 1043-1044. https://doi.org/10.1038/2151043a0

Guest, W. C., Plotkin, S. S., & Cashman, N. R. (2011). Toward a Mechanism of Prion Misfolding and Structural Models of PrPSc: Current Knowledge and Future Directions. *Journal of Toxicology and Environmental Health, Part A, 74*(2–4), 154–160.

Halfmann, R., Jarosz, D., Jones, S. et al. (2012). Prions are a common mechanism for phenotypic inheritance in wild yeasts. *Nature* 482, 363–368. https://doi.org/10.1038/nature10875

Hamir, A. N., Cutlip, R. C., Miller, J. M., Williams, E. S., Stack, M. J., Miller, M. W., O'Rourke, K. I., & Chaplin, M. J. (2001). Preliminary Findings on the Experimental Transmission of Chronic Wasting Disease Agent of Mule Deer to Cattle. *Journal of Veterinary Diagnostic Investigation, 13*(1), 91–96. https://doi.org/10.1177/104063870101300121

Hendricks, B. (2019, February 24). *Yale professor refutes popular CWD theory.* Arkansas Online. https://www.arkansasonline.com/news/2019/feb/24/yale-professor-refutes-popular-cwd-theo/.

Hsiao, K., Baker, H. F., Crow, T. J., Poulter, M., Owen, F., Terwilliger, J. D., Westaway, D., Ott, J., & Prusiner, S. B. (1989). Linkage of a prion protein missense variant to Gerstmann-Sträussler syndrome. *Nature, 338*(6213), 342–345. https://doi.org/10.1038/338342a0

Hsiao, K., Scott, M., Foster, D., Groth, D., Dearmond, S., & Prusiner, S. (1990). Spontaneous neurodegeneration in transgenic mice with mutant prion protein. *Science, 250*(4987), 1587-1590. doi:10.1126/science.1980379

http://csu-cvmbs.colostate.edu/academics/mip/prion-research-center/Pages/Prion-Basics.aspx

Huang, Z., Gabriel, J. M., Baldwin, M. A., Fletterick, R. J., Prusiner, S. B., & Cohen, F. E. (1994). Proposed three-dimensional structure for the cellular prion protein. *Proceedings of the National Academy of Sciences, 91*(15), 7139-7143. doi:10.1073/pnas.91.15.7139

Hughes, D., & Halliday, M. (2017). What Is Our Current Understanding of PrPSc-Associated Neurotoxicity and Its Molecular Underpinnings? *Pathogens, 6*(4). https://doi.org/10.3390/pathogens6040063

Imran, M., & Mahmood, S. (2011). An overview of human prion diseases. *Virology Journal, 8*, 559. https://doi.org/10.1186/1743-422X-8-559

Imran, M., & Mahmood, S. (2011). An overview of human prion diseases. *Virology Journal, 8*(1). doi:10.1186/1743-422x-8-559

Ishikura, N., Clever, J. L., Bouzamondo-Bernstein, E., Samayoa, E., Prusiner, S. B., Huang, E. J., & DeArmond, S. J. (2005). Notch-1 activation and dendritic atrophy in prion disease. *Proceedings of the National Academy of Sciences of the United States of America, 102*(3), 886–891. https://doi.org/10.1073/pnas.0408612101

Iyer, S. (2004, November 17). *Infection by Protein: The Prion Theory of Disease.* Journal of Young Investigators. https://www.jyi.org/2004-november/2017/10/17/infection-by-protein-the-prion-theory-of-disease#. (ISSN)1539-4026

John Hopkins Medicine (n.d.). Prion diseases. https://www.hopkinsmedicine.org/health/conditions-and-diseases/prion-diseases

Kahn, S., Dubé, C., Bates, L., & Balachandran, A. (2004). Chronic wasting disease in Canada: Part 1. *The Canadian Veterinary Journal, 45*(5), 397–404. https://www.ncbi.nlm.nih.gov/pmc/articles/PMC548623/

Kaneko, K., Vey, M., Scott, M., Pilkuhn, S., Cohen, F. E., & Prusiner, S. B. (1997).

COOH-terminal sequence of the cellular prion protein directs subcellular trafficking and controls conversion into the scrapie isoform. *Proceedings of the National Academy of Sciences, 94*(6), 2333-2338. doi:10.1073/pnas.94.6.2333

Karamujić-Čomić, H., Ahmad, S., Lysen, T. S., Heshmatollah, A., Roshchupkin, G. V., Vernooij, M. W., . . . Duijn, C. M. (2020). Prion protein codon 129 polymorphism in mild cognitive impairment and dementia: The Rotterdam Study. *Brain Communications, 2*(1). doi:10.1093/braincomms/fcaa030

Kim, S. H., Yu, M. M., & Strutt, A. M. (2019). Variably protease-sensitive prionopathy. *Neurology: Clinical Practice, 9*(2), 145-151. doi:10.1212/cpj.0000000000000612

Knight, R., & Collins, S. (2000). Human Prion Diseases: Cause, Clinical and Diagnostic Aspects. *Prions Contributions to Microbiology,* 68-92. doi:10.1159/000060377

Kobayashi, A., Kitamoto, T., & Mizusawa, H. (2018). Iatrogenic Creutzfeldt-Jakob disease. *Handbook of Clinical Neurology, 153*, 207–218. https://doi.org/10.1016/B978-0-444-63945-5.00012-X

Kohn, W. G., Collins, A. S., Cleveland, J. L., Harte, J. A., Eklund, K. J., & Malvitz, D. M. (2003). *Guidelines for Infection Control in Dental Health-Care Settings.* Centers for Disease Control and Prevention.

Lanska, D. J. (2018, May). Stanley Prusiner on the Origin of the Term Prion. *World Neurology: The Official Newsletter of the World Federation of Neurology.* Retrieved from: https://worldneurologyonline.com/article/stanley-prusiner-on-the-origin-of-the-term-prion/

Lanska, D. J., & Klaffke, L. E. (2017, April 27). Interview with Doctor Stanley B. Prusiner [Interview by D. J. Lanksa & L. E. Klaffke]. *The American Academy of Neurology Oral History Project at the Boston Convention & Exhibition Center,* Boston, Massachusetts. Retrieved from: https://www.aan.com/siteassets/home-page/footer/about-the-aan/history/prusiner-interview.pdf

Ledford, H. (2007). Virus paper reignites prion spat. *Nature, 445*(7128), 575. http://dx.doi.org/10.1038/445575a

Legname, G. (2017, August 31). *Elucidating the function of the prion protein.* PLOS Pathogens. https://journals.plos.org/plospathogens/article?id=10.1371%2Fjournal.ppat.1006458#:~:text=Defining%20PrP%20function%20may%20shed,a%20protective%20role%20against%20stress.

Letters, S., Smith, A. J., McHugh, S., & Bagg, J. (2005). A study of visual and blood contamination on reprocessed endodontic files from general dental practice. *British Dental Journal, 199*(8), 522–525. https://doi.org/10.1038/sj.bdj.4812811

Liberski, P. P., Gajos, A., Sikorska, B., & Lindenbaum, S. (2019). Kuru, the First Human Prion Disease. *Viruses, 11*(3), 232. https://doi.org/10.3390/v11030232

Liu, P. A. (2011). *Creating Controversy: Science Writers, Corporate Funders, and Non-expert Scientists in the Debate over Prions (1982-1997)* (dissertation). University of Toronto, Toronto.

Lledo, P. M., Tremblay, P., Dearmond, S. J., Prusiner, S. B., & Nicoll, R. A. (1996). Mice deficient for prion protein exhibit normal neuronal excitability and synaptic transmission in the hippocampus. *Proceedings of the National Academy of Sciences, 93*(6), 2403-2407. doi:10.1073/pnas.93.6.2403

Llewelyn, C., Hewitt, P., Knight, R., Amar, K., Cousens, S., Mackenzie, J., & Will, R. (2004). Possible transmission of variant Creutzfeldt-Jakob disease by blood transfusion. *The Lancet, 363*(9407), 417–421. https://doi.org/10.1016/s0140-6736(04)15486-x

Mabbott, N. A. (2012). Prion pathogenesis and secondary lymphoid organs (SLO). *Prion, 6*(4), 322–333. https://doi.org/10.4161/pri.20676

Mackenzie, G., & Will, R. (2017). Creutzfeldt-Jakob disease: Recent developments. *F1000Research, 6.* https://doi.org/10.12688/f1000research.12681.1

Mad Cow Disease: Symptoms, Causes and Treatments for vCJD. (n.d.). Retrieved from https://www.webmd.com/brain/mad-cow-disease-basics

Mathews, J., Glasse, R., & Lindenbaum, S. (1968). Kuru and Cannibalism. *The Lancet, 292*(7565), 449–452. https://doi.org/10.1016/S0140-6736(68)90482-0

McKhann, G. (2014). The Long and Winding Road: Review: *Madness and Memory: The Discovery of Prions--A New Biological Principle of Disease.* The Dana Foundation. Retrieved from: http://www.ncbi.nlm.nih.gov/pmc/articles/pmc4445594/

Mead, S., Whitfield, J., Poulter, M., Shah, P., Uphill, J., Beck, J., Campbell, T., Al-Dujaily, H., Hummerich, H., Alpers, M. P., & Collinge, J. (2008). Genetic susceptibility, evolution and the kuru epidemic. *Philosophical Transactions of the Royal Society B: Biological Sciences, 363*(1510), 3741–3746. https://doi.org/10.1098/rstb.2008.0087

Meiner, Z., Gabizon, R., & Prusiner, S. B. (1997). Familial Creutzfeldt-Jakob disease. Codon 200 prion disease in Libyan Jews. *Medicine, 76*(4), 227–237. https://doi.org/10.1097/00005792-199707000-00001

Michelitsch, M. D., & Weissman, J. S. (2000). A census of glutamine/asparagine-rich regions: Implications for their conserved function and the prediction of novel prions. *Proceedings of the National Academy of Sciences, 97*(22), 11910-11915. doi:10.1073/pnas.97.22.11910

Milhavet, O., McMahon, H. E. M., Rachidi, W., Nishida, N., Katamine, S., Mangé, A., Arlotto, M., Casanova, D., Riondel, J., Favier, A., & Lehmann, S. (2000). Prion infection impairs the cellular response to oxidative stress. *Proceed-*

ings of the National Academy of Sciences, 97(25), 13937–13942. https://doi.org/10.1073/pnas.250289197

Naslavsky, N., Stein, R., Yanai, A., Friedlander, G., & Taraboulos, A. (1997). Characterization of Detergent-insoluble Complexes Containing the Cellular Prion Protein and Its Scrapie Isoform. *Journal of Biological Chemistry, 272*(10), 6324-6331. doi:10.1074/jbc.272.10.6324

Nishimura, Y., Harada, K., Koyama, T., Hagiya, H., & Otsuka, F. (2020). A nationwide trend analysis in the incidence and mortality of Creutzfeldt–Jakob disease in Japan between 2005 and 2014. *Scientific Reports, 10*(1), 15509. https://doi.org/10.1038/s41598-020-72519-0

Occurrence and Transmission | Creutzfeldt-Jakob Disease, Classic (CJD) | Prion Disease | CDC. (2021, January 13). Centers for Disease Control and Prevention. https://www.cdc.gov/prions/cjd/occurrence-transmission.html

Pan, K. M., Baldwin, M., Nguyen, J., Gasset, M., Serban, A., Groth, D., Mehlhorn, I., Huang, Z., Fletterick, R. J., & Cohen, F. E. (1993). Conversion of alpha-helices into beta-sheets features in the formation of the scrapie prion proteins. *Proceedings of the National Academy of Sciences, 90*(23), 10962-10966. doi:10.1073/pnas.90.23.10962

Pedersen, N. S., & Smith, E. (2002). Prion diseases: Epidemiology in man. *APMIS: Acta Pathologica, Microbiologica, et Immunologica Scandinavica, 110*(1), 14–22. https://doi.org/10.1034/j.1600-0463.2002.100103.x

Penn University Archives and Records Center. (n.d.). *Penn People: Britton Chance 1913-2010.* University Archives and Records Center. Retrieved from: https://archives.upenn.edu/exhibits/penn-people/biography/britton-chance

Perutz, M. F., Johnson, T. T., Suzuki, M. U., & Finch, J. U. (1994). Glutamine repeats as polar zippers: Their possible role in inherited neurodegenerative diseases. *Proceedings of the National Academy of Sciences, 91*(12), 5355-5358. doi:10.1073/pnas.91.12.5355

Peters, P. J., Mironov, A., Peretz, D., Donselaar, E. V., Leclerc, E., Erpel, S., Prusiner, S. B. (2003). Trafficking of prion proteins through a caveolae-mediated endosomal pathway. *Journal of Cell Biology, 162*(4), 703-717. doi:10.1083

Pöschel, T., Brilliantov, N. V., & Frömmel, C. (2003). Kinetics of Prion Growth. *Biophysical Journal, 85*(6), 3460–3474.

Prasad, K. N., & Bondy, S. C. (2018). Oxidative and Inflammatory Events in Prion Diseases: Can they Be Therapeutic Targets? *Current Aging Science, 11*(4), 216–225. https://doi.org/10.2174/1874609812666190111100205

Priola, S. A. (2003). *BIOMEDICINE: A View from the Top--Prion Diseases from 10,000 Feet.* https://doi.org/10.1126/science.1085920

PRNP gene. (2020, August 18). Retrieved from https://medlineplus.gov/genetics/
  g e n e / p r n p / PRNP prion protein [Homo sapiens (human)]. (n.d.).
  Retrieved from https://www.ncbi.nlm.nih.gov/gene/5621

Prusiner, S. (1991). Molecular biology of prion diseases. *Science, 252*(5012), 1515-1522.
  doi:10.1126/science.1675487

Prusiner, S. B. (1984). Some Speculations about Prions, Amyloid, and Alzheimers
  Disease. *New England Journal of Medicine, 310*(10), 661-663. doi:10.1056/
  nejm198403083101021

Prusiner, S. B. (1997). *Stanley B. Prusiner Biographical.* Retrieved from https://www.
  nobelprize.org/prizes/medicine/1997/prusiner/biographical/

Prusiner, S. B. (1998). Prions. *Proc. Natl. Acad. Sc. USA (PNAS), 95*, 13363-13383.
  https://doi.org/10.1073/pnas.95.23.13363

Prusiner, S. B. (2014). *Madness and Memory: The Discovery of Prions--A New Biological
  Principle of Disease.* Yale University Press.

Prusiner, S. B., Scott, M., Foster, D., Pan, K., Groth, D., Mirenda, C., Torchia, M.,
  Yang, S. L., Serban, D., Carlson, G. A., Peter, C. H., Westway, D., Dearmond, S. J. (1990). Transgenetic studies implicate interactions between
  homologous PrP isoforms in scrapie prion replication. *Cell, 63*(4), 673-686.
  doi:10.1016/0092-8674(90)90134-z

Qina, T., Sanjo, N., Hizume, M., Higuma, M., Tomita, M., Atarashi, R., . . . Mizusawa,
  H. (2014). Clinical features of genetic Creutzfeldt-Jakob disease with V180I
  mutation in the prion protein gene. *BMJ Open, 4*(5). doi:10.1136/bmjop-
  en-2014-004968

Rambaran, R. N., & Serpell, L. C. (2008). Amyloid fibrils. *Prion, 2*(3), 112–117.
  https://doi.org/10.4161/pri.2.3.7488

Raymond, G. J. (2000). Evidence of a molecular barrier limiting susceptibility of
  humans, cattle and sheep to chronic wasting disease. *The EMBO Journal,
  19*(17), 4425–4430. https://doi.org/10.1093/emboj/19.17.4425

Robertson, S. (2021, April 15). *What is a prion?* Medical News. https://www.
  news-medical.net/health/What-is-a-Prion.aspx

Saba, R., & Booth, S. A. (2013). The Genetics of Susceptibility to Variant
  Creutzfeldt-Jakob Disease. *Public Health Genomics, 16*(1–2), 17–24. https://
  doi.org/10.1159/000345203

Sajnani, G., & Requena, J. R. (2012). Prions, proteinase K and infectivity. *Prion, 6*(5),
  430–432. https://doi.org/10.4161/pri.22309

Saunders, S. E., Bartelt-Hunt, S. L., & Bartz, J. C. (2008). Prions in the environment.
  Prion, 2(4), 162–169.

Scheckel, C., & Aguzzi, A. (2018). Prions, prionoids and protein misfolding disorders. *Nature Reviews Genetics, 19*(7), 405–418. https://doi.org/10.1038/s41576-018-0011-4

Scientific American. (1999, October 21). *What is a prion?: The molecular structure of prions and how they cause infections like Creutzfeldt-Jakob disease.* https://www.scientificamerican.com/article/what-is-a-prion-specifica/

Senatore, A., Restelli, E., & Chiesa, R. (2013). Synaptic Dysfunction in Prion Diseases: A Trafficking Problem? *International Journal of Cell Biology, 2013,* e543803. https://doi.org/10.1155/2013/543803

Shkundina, I. S., & Ter-Avanesyan, M. D. (2007). Prions. *Biochemistry (Moscow), 72*(13), 1519-1536. doi:10.1134/s0006297907130081

Sigurðsson, B. (1954). RIDA, a chronic encephalitis of sheep: With general remarks on infections which develop slowly and some of their special characteristics. *British Veterinary Journal, 110*(9), 341-354. https://doi.org/10.1016/S0007-1935(17)50172-4

Smith, A. J., Bagg, J., Ironside, J. W., Will, R. G., & Scully, C. (2003). Prions and the oral cavity. *Journal of Dental Research, 82*(10), 769–775. https://doi.org/10.1177/154405910308201002

Smith, A., Dickson, M., Aitken, J., & Bagg, J. (2002). Contaminated dental instruments. *Journal of Hospital Infection, 51*(3), 233–235. https://doi.org/10.1053/jhin.2002.1213

Smith, P. G., & Bradley, R. (2003). Bovine spongiform encephalopathy (BSE) and its epidemiology. *British Medical Bulletin, 66*(1), 185–198. https://doi.org/10.1093/bmb/66.1.185

Sorensen, S. (2019, March 7). *Bacteria and CWD Cure: Dr. Bastian Speaks.* Deer and Deer Hunting. https://www.deeranddeerhunting.com/content/articles/deer-news/bacteria-and-cwd-cure-dr-bastian-speaks.

Soto, C. (2011, March). *Prion hypothesis: The end of the controversy?* https://doi.org/10.1016/j.tibs.2010.11.001

Soto, C., & Satani, N. (2011). The intricate mechanisms of neurodegeneration in prion diseases. *Trends in Molecular Medicine, 17*(1), 14–24. https://doi.org/10.1016/j.molmed.2010.09.001

Stahl, N. (1987). Scrapie prion protein contains a phosphatidylinositol glycolipid. *Cell, 51*(2), 229-240. doi:10.1016/0092-8674(87)90150-

Stahl, N., Baldwin, M. A., Teplow, D. B., Hood, L., Gibson, B. W., Burlingame, A. L., & Prusiner, S. B. (1993). Structural studies of the scrapie prion protein using mass spectrometry and amino acid sequencing. *Biochemistry, 32*(8), 1991-2002. doi:10.1021/bi00059a016

Surveillance for vCJD | Variant Creutzfeldt-Jakob Disease, Classic (CJD) | Prion Disease |
    CDC. (2019, October 24). Centers for Disease Control and Prevention.
    https://www.cdc.gov/prions/vcjd/surveillance.html

Sushma, B., Gugwad, S., Pavaskar, R., & Malik, S. A. (2016). Prions in dentistry: A
    need to be concerned and known. *Journal of Oral and Maxillofacial Pathology :
    JOMFP, 20*(1), 111–114. https://doi.org/10.4103/0973-029X.180961

Tanford, C., & Reynolds, J. (2001). *Nature's Robots: A History of Proteins.* St Ives: Ox-
    ford University Press. [   ]

Taubes, Gary. (1986). *The game of the name is fame. But is it science?* Discover, 28-52

Taylor, D. M. (1999). Inactivation of prions by physical and chemical means. *Journal
    of Hospital Infection, 43*(Suppl. 1), S69–S76. https://doi.org/10.1016/s0195-
    6701(99)90067-1

Telling G.C. (2013). The importance of prions. *PLoS pathogens, 9*(1), e1003090.
    https://doi.org/10.1371/journal.ppat.1003090

Telling, G. C., Scott, M., Hsiao, K. K., Foster, D., Yang, S. L., Torchia, M., Sidle, K.
    C., Collinge, J., DeArmond, S. J., & Prusiner, S. B. (1994). Transmission
    of Creutzfeldt-Jakob disease from humans to transgenic mice expressing
    chimeric human-mouse prion protein. *Proceedings of the National Academy of
    Sciences, 91*(21), 9936-9940. doi:10.1073/pnas.91.21.9936

Telling, G. C., Scott, M., Mastrianni, J., Gabizon, R., Torchia, M., Cohen, F. E.,
    DeArmond, S. J., & Prusiner, S. B. (1995). Prion propagation in mice
    expressing human and chimeric PrP transgenes implicates the interaction
    of cellular PrP with another protein. *Cell, 83*(1), 79-90. doi:10.1016/0092-
    8674(95)90236-8

The Independent . (2007, May 20). *Mark Purdey.* Mark Purdey - Independent Online
    Edition > Obituaries. https://web.archive.org/web/20070520193755/
    http://news.independent.co.uk/people/obituaries/article1990371.ece.

Tittelmeier, J., Nachman, E., & Nussbaum-Krammer, C. (2020). Molecular Chaper-
    ones: A Double-Edged Sword in Neurodegenerative Diseases. *Frontiers in
    Aging Neuroscience*, 12, 321. https://doi.org/10.3389/fnagi.2020.581374

Tremblay, P., Ball, H. L., Kaneko, K., Groth, D., Hegde, R. S., Cohen, F. E., DeAr-
    mond, S. J., Prusiner, S. B., & Safar, J. G. (2004). Mutant PrPSc Conformers
    Induced by a Synthetic Peptide and Several Prion Strains. *Journal of Virology,
    78*(4), 2088-2099. doi:10.1128/jvi.78.4.2088-2099.2004

U. S. Food and Drug Administration/Center for Biologics Evaluation and Research.
    (2010) *Revised Preventive Measures to Reduce the Possible Risk of Transmission of
    Creutzfeldt-Jakob Disease and Variant Creutzfeldt-Jakob Disease by Blood and Blood
    Products.* Author.

Urayama, A., Concha-Marambio, L., Khan, U., Bravo-Alegria, J., Kharat, V., & Soto, C. (2016). *Scientific Reports, 6*(1), 32338. https://doi.org/10.1038/srep32338

Vey, M., Pilkuhn, S., Wille, H., Nixon, R., Dearmond, S. J., Smart, E. J., Anderson, R. G. W., Taraboulos, A., & Prusiner, S. B. (1996). Subcellular colocalization of the cellular and scrapie prion proteins in caveolae-like membranous domains. *Proceedings of the National Academy of Sciences, 93*(25), 14945-14949. doi:10.1073/pnas.93.25.14945

Westaway, D., Goodman, P. A., Mirenda, C. A., Mckinley, M. P., Carlson, G. A., & Prusiner, S. B. (1987). Distinct prion proteins in short and long scrapie incubation period mice. *Cell, 51*(4), 651-662. doi:10.1016/0092-8674(87)90134-6

Westergard, L., Christensen, H. M., & Harris, D. A. (2007). The Cellular Prion Protein (PrPC): Its Physiological Function and Role in Disease. *Biochimica et Biophysica Acta, 1772*(6), 629–644. https://doi.org/10.1016/j.bbadis.2007.02.011

Whittington, M. A., Sidle, K. C., Gowland, I., Meads, J., Hill, A. F., Palmer, M. S., Jefferys, J. G. R., & Collinge, J. (1995). Rescue of neurophysiological phenotype seen in PrP null mice by transgene encoding human prion protein. *Nature Genetics, 9*(2), 197-201. doi:10.1038/ng0295-197

Wickner, R. B. (1994). [URE3] as an altered URE2 protein: evidence for a prion analog in Saccharomyces cerevisiae. *Science*, 264(5158), 566-569. https://doi.org/10.1126/science.7909170

Wille, H., & Requena, J. R. (2018, February 7). *The Structure of PrPSc Prions*. Pathogens (Basel, Switzerland). https://www.ncbi.nlm.nih.gov/pmc/articles/PMC5874746/ doi:10.3390/pathogens7010020.

Yegya-Raman, N., Aziz, R., Schneider, D., Tobia, A., Leitch, M., & Nwobi, O. (2018). Corrigendum to "A Case of Sporadic Creutzfeldt-Jakob Disease Presenting as Conversion Disorder." *Case Reports in Psychiatry, 2018*, e3826863. https://doi.org/10.1155/2018/3826863

Zabel, M. D., & Reid, C. (2015). A brief history of prions. *Pathogens and Disease, 73*(9). https://dx.doi.org/10.1093%2Ffemspd%2Fftv087

www.ingramcontent.com/pod-product-compliance
Lightning Source LLC
Chambersburg PA
CBHW071750270326
41928CB00013B/2862